GASTRITIS
Foods, Supplements & Herbs

Isabel M. Rivero

COPYRIGHT & CREDITS

GASTRITIS. Foods, Supplements & Herbs.
Copyright©2017, 2024 *by* Isabel M. Rivero
All rights reserved

Without limiting the rights reserved under copyright law, no part of this book may be reproduced, distributed, stored in a retrieval system, or transmitted in any form or by any means, whether electronic, mechanical, photocopying, recording, or otherwise, without prior written permission from the author.

Thank you for respecting this work. By supporting original publications and avoiding piracy, you help ensure the creation of new ebooks in the future. Your collaboration allows authors and publishers to continue bringing valuable content to readers.

Cover design: Valeria Veretennikova & Desirée Mendoza M.
Photographs by Buntysmum and Nidan via Pixabay

This book provides general information and is not a substitute for professional medical advice. Neither the publisher nor the author shall be held liable for any damages of any kind arising from the use of this content. Readers assume full responsibility for their decisions, actions, and outcomes.

This book is intended as a reference only and should never be used as a medical manual. Its purpose is to help readers make informed decisions about their health. It is not intended to replace any treatment prescribed by a doctor.

Original title: *GASTRITIS. Alimentos y Plantas Medicinales* © 2017, Isabel M. Rivero. All Rights Reserved
© 2024 translated by Sara I. Afonso & Laura Mendoza

Prologue: A Guide to Wellness

Dear Readers,

Welcome to this journey toward better health! Since I began sharing my knowledge and experience, my primary motivation has been to make a positive contribution to your lives. That's why, through these pages, I aim to offer valuable information and practical resources that can genuinely help you feel better.

In this book, every piece of advice and remedy has been thoughtfully chosen for its proven effectiveness and practicality in everyday life. You will discover not only medicinal plants, supplements, and accessible foods but also detailed medical insights into this health concern, along with additional tips and answers to the most frequently asked questions–providing you with a practical, comprehensive, and trustworthy guide.

My goal is for this work to be your valuable and practical companion–a resource where you can find tangible tools to support you on your journey toward a healthier, more fulfilling life. Knowing that this work has a positive impact brings me great joy and motivates me to keep going. While writing requires effort, time, and perseverance, the knowledge that my books make a meaningful difference in your lives is my greatest reward.

Because your experiences are my greatest source of inspiration, I would love for you to write to me and share your progress. Feel free to share your progress by writing directly to me at **isabelmriveror@gmail.com**. Your stories inspire me and truly make my efforts worthwhile.

I sincerely hope this practical guide becomes your indispensable pillar on your journey to better health and well-being. Thank you for allowing me to be part of your life.

With love,

                    Isabel

INTRODUCTION

On our journey toward optimal health, it's essential to understand that no "miracle" remedy–whether it's a medication, herb, supplement, or food–can fully address an illness on its own. Similarly, focusing solely on alleviating symptoms without addressing the underlying "cause" increases the risk of relapse. Treating the root of the problem, however, gradually reduces symptoms and promotes true and lasting recovery.

You may have noticed that, at times, medications don't work as expected. This happens because regaining health requires a holistic treatment approach that addresses the actual cause of the problem at its root. In addition to effective treatments, this approach should include changes in diet, sleep quality, stress management, and overall lifestyle habits.

With this book, we will explore a holistic approach to health. In the first chapter, you'll find key information to help you understand the main causes of this disease, along with its symptoms, types, warning signs, common complications, helpful advice, and the essential medical tests needed for an accurate diagnosis. In the following chapters, we'll dive into strategies to support recovery, including dietary guidance, daily menus, and natural approaches such as supplements and herbal remedies for gradual improvement.

While you can independently choose your preferred remedies, the chapter "**Suggested Practical Plan**" will serve as your primary guide. This section offers a comprehensive approach, addressing all essential aspects of recovery. From there, you'll be directed to other chapters and can apply the recommendations best suited to your unique situation.

It's important to emphasize that the benefits of the recommendations provided in this book are grounded in scientific evidence, rather than personal opinions. At the end, you'll find references and studies supporting each remedy, ensuring you feel confident and secure when applying them.

GASTRITIS

The stomach is nothing short of a marvel–a vital organ in the digestive system that works tirelessly every day to break down the food we eat and transform it into the nutrients our bodies depend on to thrive. Tucked between the esophagus and the small intestine, the stomach acts as a dynamic, muscular chamber, powerfully churning food into a smooth, digestible mixture aided by potent gastric acids. While it may seem at first glance like a hostile environment–filled with corrosive hydrochloric acid (HCl) and sharp digestive enzymes like pepsin –the stomach is equipped with finely tuned defense mechanisms to ensure it maintains the delicate balance required for its intricate function.

At the heart of this remarkable system lies the gastric mucosa: a protective layer of tissue that acts as a shield, safeguarding the stomach lining from damage caused by its own powerful acids and enzymes. This mucosa produces a thick, protective coating of mucus enriched with bicarbonate to neutralize harmful acids, while the stomach's tight cellular structure and robust blood flow maintain its health and ability to repair itself. Yet, this masterfully orchestrated system is surprisingly fragile, dependent on a careful equilibrium between protective forces and potentially destructive ones.

When this balance tips–from excessive acid production, infection by Helicobacter pylori, chronic stress, overuse of nonsteroidal anti-inflammatory drugs (NSAIDs), or alcohol consumption–the gastric mucosa becomes compromised. As the protective barrier weakens, stomach acid and enzymes penetrate deeper into the tissue, triggering inflammation and damage–this is the condition we know as gastritis.

On a deeper, cellular level, gastritis sets off an immune response as the body tries to repair itself. Specialized cells in the stomach release inflammatory chemicals like cytokines and histamines, which, while aimed at healing, often exacerbate irritation and swelling in the mucosa. Left unchecked, this chronic inflammation can progress, manifesting symptoms like burning pain in the upper abdomen, nausea, bloating, indigestion, or even loss of appetite. And if neglected or poorly managed, the consequences can escalate–complications such as ulcers, gastrointestinal bleeding, and, in severe cases, an increased risk of developing stomach cancer.

Gastritis is far more than a simple medical condition; it is a deeply disruptive force that affects millions of lives around the world. Beyond the physical discomfort–like pain and nausea–it profoundly influences day-to-day living. Deciding what to eat becomes stressful. Plans and routines are reshaped. Energy levels drop. Quality of life often diminishes as people grapple with frustration and a sense of helplessness in their search for relief.

The encouraging news? Real solutions are within reach. By understanding how the stomach works, what throws it off balance, and how that balance can be restored, you can find not just relief, but a path to long-term well-being. That's what this book is all about. It's designed to be your guide–a resource for anyone who has wrestled with the challenges of gastritis and seeks not just to manage the condition, but to reclaim their quality of life. Together, we'll delve into the powerful role of diet, stress reduction, and avoiding irritants like alcohol or NSAIDs in helping your stomach heal and stay healthy.

But beyond all else, this book is about empowering you. Whether you've recently been diagnosed with gastritis, have struggled with it for years, or simply seek to protect your digestive health, within these pages you'll find practical guidance, natural remedies, and insights that work in harmony with your body's natural ability to heal. From uncovering the root causes of gastritis to exploring strategies and treatments that calm, strengthen, and restore, this journey is about much more than managing a stomach condition–it's about reclaiming balance, not only in your digestive system but in your overall well-being.

You are not alone in this journey. Millions of people face the challenges of gastritis every day, and many have taken the same first steps toward relief and recovery. This book will be your companion, offering you not only knowledge but also hope and encouragement. Together, we'll navigate the path toward healing, comfort, and a better quality of life.

This is your moment to take charge of your health and start making meaningful changes. You are capable of achieving relief and restoring balance, and you deserve to live free from the discomfort of gastritis. The journey begins here–let's take that first step together.

Symptoms

Gastritis can manifest in a variety of ways, with symptoms that differ in intensity and frequency. These discomforts may appear suddenly as acute episodes or develop gradually, turning into a chronic condition. Recognizing these symptoms is crucial for understanding how this condition impacts the body. The most common symptoms are outlined below:

▸ **Abdominal pain**: Abdominal pain is among the most common gastritis symptoms. It can vary in intensity and location and is commonly described as a burning sensation, tightness, or discomfort in the upper abdomen. The pain may worsen after eating, especially if irritating or fatty foods are consumed.

▸ **Heartburn**: Heartburn, also known as reflux, is a burning sensation or discomfort in the chest that occurs when stomach acid refluxes into the esophagus. This symptom may be present in gastritis due to increased stomach acid production or decreased protection of the gastric lining.

▸ **Nausea and vomiting**: Many individuals with gastritis experience nausea and, in some cases, vomiting. These symptoms may be caused by gastric lining irritation, acid in the stomach, or decreased gastric motility.

▸ **Loss of appetite**: Gastritis can cause a decreased appetite, leading to reduced food intake. If not adequately treated, this can result in unintentional weight loss and malnutrition.

- **Feeling of fullness or early satiety**: Some people with gastritis may experience a feeling of fullness or early satiety, meaning they feel full after eating only a tiny amount. This can lead to decreased food intake and weight loss.

- **Abdominal bloating**: Gastritis can cause abdominal bloating or distention, making the abdomen feel full and tight. This can be uncomfortable and affect the quality of life.

- **Changes in bowel movements**: In some cases, gastritis can cause changes in bowel movement patterns. These symptoms may include diarrhea or constipation and vary in intensity and duration.

- **Fatigue and weakness**: Chronic inflammation in the stomach can affect the absorption of essential nutrients, leading to a deficiency of vitamins and minerals. This can result in fatigue, weakness, and lack of energy.

- **Gastrointestinal bleeding**: In some cases of gastritis, gastrointestinal bleeding may occur when the stomach lining is eroded or ulcerated. This may manifest as vomiting blood or material similar to coffee grounds or black, tarry stools (melena stools). Gastrointestinal bleeding requires immediate and urgent medical attention, as it may signify a more severe illness.

- **Bad breath**: Chronic gastritis can cause persistent bad breath. This may be caused by bacteria in the stomach that produce volatile sulfur compounds, which generate an unpleasant odor.

- **Feeling of general malaise**: Some people may experience a feeling of general malaise, such as fatigue, weakness, irritability, or generalized body discomfort.

- **Chest pain**: Some people with gastritis may experience chest pain similar to the pain associated with a heart attack. The symptoms can be similar, making this condition confusing and worrisome. It is important to mention any chest pain to a physician to rule out other potentially serious conditions, such as a heart attack.

▸ **Frequent belching**: Gastritis can cause increased gas production in the stomach, leading to frequent belching. Due to stomach acid reflux, these burps may taste sour or bitter.

▸ **Burning sensation in the mouth or throat**: Some people with gastritis may experience a burning sensation in the mouth or throat, known as mouth burning or pharyngeal burning. This may be caused by stomach acid reflux into the esophagus and mouth.

▸ **Stomach tenderness**: In cases of acute gastritis, the stomach area may be tender to the touch. Gently pressing on the abdomen may cause discomfort or pain.

▸ **Appetite changes**: Gastritis can affect appetite and taste for food. Some people may experience a decreased appetite, while others crave acidic or spicy foods. There may also be a feeling of early satiety after eating even small amounts of food.

▸ **Nighttime discomfort**: Some people may experience gastritis symptoms, such as abdominal pain or heartburn, especially at night or bedtime. This may be due to the horizontal position, which facilitates acid reflux from the stomach into the esophagus.

It is essential to consider that gastritis symptoms can vary from person to person and, in many cases, resemble those of other gastrointestinal conditions.

Types

Gastritis is categorized into various types, each distinguished by its unique features and specific causes. The most notable types include the following:

▸ **Acute gastritis**: This type of gastritis develops suddenly and lasts for a short duration. It can be caused by bacterial infections, such as Helicobacter pylori bacteria, excessive alcohol consumption, prolonged use of non-steroidal anti-inflammatory drugs (NSAIDs), or chronic stress. Typical symptoms include abdominal pain, nausea, vomiting, and loss of appetite.

▸ **Chronic gastritis**: In contrast to acute gastritis, chronic gastritis develops slowly and may persist for months or years. The most common cause of chronic gastritis is H. pylori infection, a bacterium that colonizes the stomach and causes ongoing inflammation. Other factors, such as regular alcohol consumption, bile reflux and certain autoimmune diseases, can also contribute to chronic gastritis. Symptoms can vary but often include abdominal discomfort, fullness, nausea and weight loss.

▸ **Atrophic gastritis**: This type of gastritis is characterized by chronic inflammation of the stomach lining, which decreases acid-producing cells and digestive enzymes. It may be associated with H. pylori infection or autoimmune disorders, such as Biermer's disease, in which the immune system attacks gastric cells. Atrophic gastritis can cause symptoms similar to chronic gastritis and nutritional deficiencies due to mal-absorption.

▸ **Erosive gastritis**: This type causes erosions or ulcers in the stomach lining. It may be caused by excessive alcohol consumption, prolonged use of NSAIDs, bacterial infections, or other diseases. Symptoms include severe abdominal pain, gastrointestinal bleeding, nausea and vomiting.

▸ **Stress gastritis**: This type of gastritis develops after a serious illness, trauma, surgery, or severe burns. Extreme stress can affect blood flow to the stomach lining and cause inflammation. Symptoms are often similar to those of acute gastritis.

▸ **Fundic gastritis**: This form mainly affects the body region and gastric fundus, where the cells that produce hydro-chloric acid and intrinsic factors are located. Bacterial infections, autoimmune disorders, or abnormal cells in the gastric lining may cause it. Fundic gastritis can decrease the production of acid and digestive enzymes, affecting digestion and nutrient absorption.

▸ **Eosinophilic gastritis**: This type of gastritis results from an excessive accumulation of eosinophils, a type of inflammatory cell, in the stomach lining. The exact cause is not always clear, but it is thought to be related to food allergies, immune reactions, or systemic disorders. Symptoms may include abdominal pain, nausea, vomiting, difficulty swallowing, and weight loss.

▸ **Chemical gastritis**: This type occurs when the body is exposed to irritating chemicals, such as strong acids, alkalis, or certain industrial chemicals. It can result from accidental ingestion, occupational exposure, or consumption of corrosive substances. Depending on the amount and duration of exposure, symptoms can range from mild to severe and include severe abdominal pain, bloody vomiting, and difficulty swallowing.

▸ **Gastritis is associated with specific diseases**: Some diseases, such as Crohn's, celiac, and sarcoidosis, can cause inflammation in the stomach as part of their systemic manifestation. These forms of gastritis are often related to the underlying disease and may require a specific treatment approach.

▸ **Granulomatous gastritis**: This type of gastritis is characterized by the formation of granulomas in the stomach lining. Granulomas are aggregates of inflammatory cells and scar tissue that develop in response to chronic infections or systemic diseases, such as tuberculosis or Crohn's disease. Symptoms may include abdominal pain, weight loss, nausea and vomiting.

▸ **Alcoholic gastritis**: It is caused by chronic and excessive alcohol consumption, which irritates and damages the stomach lining. Alcoholic gastritis can lead to chronic inflammation, ulcers, and bleeding in the stomach. Symptoms may include abdominal pain, nausea, vomiting blood, and loss of appetite.

▸ **NSAID-induced gastritis**: Long-term use of non-steroidal anti-inflammatory drugs (NSAIDs), such as ibuprofen or naproxen, can irritate the stomach lining and cause gastritis. These drugs can decrease the production of prostaglandins, which protect the stomach, increasing the risk of inflammation and ulcers. Symptoms may include abdominal pain, heartburn, nausea and vomiting.

▸ **Postoperative gastritis**: After abdominal surgery, mainly if partial or total stomach removal (gastrectomy) was performed, gastritis may develop due to surgical stress and changes in the anatomy and function of the stomach. Symptoms can vary but may include abdominal pain, nausea, vomiting, and difficulty eating and digesting food.

▸ **Allergic gastritis**: This type of gastritis is caused by an allergic reaction to certain foods. When an allergic person consumes foods to which they are sensitive, their immune system may trigger an inflammatory response in the stomach lining. Symptoms may include abdominal pain, nausea, vomiting, diarrhea, and sometimes difficulty breathing or swelling in the body.

▸ **Radiation gastritis**: Radiation therapy to the abdominal or pelvic area as part of cancer treatment can cause damage to the stomach lining, leading to radiation gastritis. Symptoms may include abdominal pain, nausea, vomiting, diarrhea, and loss of appetite. These symptoms usually improve gradually after the end of treatment.

▸ **Infectious gastritis**: In addition to Helicobacter pylori infection, other infections can cause gastritis. Some organisms, such as herpes simplex virus, cytomegalovirus, and certain bacteria and fungi, can infect the stomach and cause inflammation. Symptoms may vary depending on the organism involved, including abdominal pain, nausea, vomiting and fever.

▸ **Drug-induced gastritis**: Some medications can cause irritation or inflammation in the stomach lining, leading to drug-induced gastritis. Common examples include certain antibiotics, corticosteroids, drugs to treat osteoporosis, and some antidepressants. Symptoms may include abdominal pain, nausea, vomiting and stomach upset.

It is essential to emphasize that accurately identifying gastritis and determining its specific type requires a thorough medical evaluation.

Causes

Gastritis can arise from various factors, and identifying its underlying cause is crucial for effective treatment. Below are the most common ones:

‣ **Helicobacter pylori infection**: The leading cause of gastritis is infection by the bacterium Helicobacter pylori (H. pylori). This bacterium is highly contagious and is transmitted mainly through contaminated food and water and by direct contact with an infected person. H. pylori attaches to the stomach lining and produces chemicals irritating and damaging gastric tissue, leading to inflammation and gastritis.

‣ **Long-term use of nonsteroidal anti-inflammatory** drugs (NSAIDs): NSAIDs, such as ibuprofen and naproxen, are commonly used to relieve pain and inflammation. However, prolonged use can irritate the stomach lining and cause gastritis. These drugs can interfere with the production of prostaglandins, chemicals that protect the stomach lining.

‣ **Excessive alcohol consumption**: Excessive and prolonged alcohol consumption can damage the stomach lining and cause gastritis. Alcohol increases stomach acid production and also weakens the stomach's protective barrier, which facilitates irritation and inflammation.

‣ **Chronic stress**: Chronic stress can trigger gastritis in some people. Prolonged stress can affect immune system function and increase stomach acid production, damaging the stomach lining and causing inflammation.

‣ **Bile reflux into the stomach**: Bile is a fluid produced by the liver that aids in the digestion of fats. In some cases, bile can back up from the intestine into the stomach, irritating and damaging the gastric lining and causing gastritis.

‣ **Autoimmune disorders**: In some cases, the immune system may mistakenly attack the stomach lining cells, known as autoimmune gastritis. This form of gastritis can be chronic and is often associated with other autoimmune diseases, such as Hashimoto's disease or type 1 diabetes.

‣ **Hereditary factors**: There is evidence that certain people may have a genetic predisposition to develop gastritis. If you have a family history of gastritis, you may have a higher risk of developing this disease.

‣ **Food irritants**: Some foods and beverages can irritate the stomach lining and trigger gastritis in some people. These foods may include spicy, acidic, fatty, fried foods, carbonated drinks, coffee and alcohol. Everyone may have different food sensitivities, so paying attention to and avoiding the foods that cause discomfort is essential.

‣ **Autoimmune disorders**: In addition to the autoimmune gastritis mentioned above, other autoimmune disorders can trigger stomach lining inflammation. Examples include Crohn's disease, celiac disease and Behçet's disease. These disorders can cause an abnormal immune response that damages gastric tissue.

‣ **Viral infections**: Although less common, some viral infections can cause gastritis. These viruses include Epstein-Barr, cytomegalovirus, and human immunodeficiency virus (HIV). Viral infection can irritate and damage the stomach lining, leading to inflammation and gastritis.

‣ **Digestive diseases**: Some digestive diseases, such as Crohn's, ulcerative colitis, and celiac disease, may be associated with gastritis. These diseases can cause chronic inflammation in the gastrointestinal tract, including the stomach.

‣ **Radiotherapy and chemotherapy**: Radiotherapy and

chemotherapy, mainly when directed to the abdominal region, can cause inflammation and damage to the stomach lining, leading to gastritis. These treatments are commonly used in people with cancer and may be necessary to fight the disease, but they can also have side effects on the digestive system.

▸ **Gastrointestinal motility disorders**: Disorders that affect the motility of the digestive system, such as irritable bowel syndrome or gastroparesis, may predispose to gastritis. These disorders can disrupt the normal movement of food through the stomach and cause a buildup of stomach acid, which increases the risk of inflammation of the stomach lining.

▸ **Autoimmune diseases**: In addition to the autoimmune gastritis mentioned above, other autoimmune diseases may be associated with gastritis. Examples include Addison's disease, systemic lupus erythematosus, and rheumatoid arthritis. These diseases can trigger an abnormal immune response that damages gastric tissue and causes inflammation.

▸ **Coagulation disorders**: Some coagulation disorders, such as idiopathic thrombocytopenic purpura or hemophilia, may increase the risk of developing gastritis. Impaired blood clotting can result in bleeding in the stomach, which irritates the lining and triggers inflammation.

▸ **Endocrine disorders**: Some endocrine disorders, such as hypothyroidism or Cushing's disease, may predispose to gastritis. Hormonal imbalances associated with these disorders can affect stomach function and increase the risk of inflammation of the gastric lining.

▸ **Genetic factors**: Certain genes have been suggested to increase the susceptibility to developing gastritis. These genetic factors may influence the immune system response, stomach acid production, and the integrity of the gastric lining.

If you experience persistent or concerning gastritis symptoms, it is vital to consult a healthcare professional for an accurate diagnosis and a personalized treatment plan. A physician can assess your symptoms, conduct necessary tests, and identify the specific cause of your gastritis to guide you toward effective relief and recovery.

Possible Long-Term Complications

This section is designed to offer clear guidance and effectively highlight potential risks, with an emphasis on prevention. By doing so, you can take proactive steps to safeguard your well-being and minimize the likelihood of complications.

The primary complications that may develop as a result of untreated gastritis are outlined below.

▸ **Ulcers**: Chronic gastritis, mainly if caused by Helicobacter pylori infection or long-term use of nonsteroidal anti-inflammatory drugs (NSAIDs), can increase the risk of developing ulcers in the stomach or duodenum (the first part of the small intestine). Ulcers are open wounds in the lining of the stomach or duodenum that can cause abdominal pain, bleeding and perforation. If left untreated, ulcers can lead to severe complications, such as internal bleeding or perforation of the organ.

▸ **Anemia**: Chronic gastritis can affect the absorption of iron and vitamin B12 in the stomach. Lack of these essential nutrients can lead to anemia, in which the body does not produce enough healthy red blood cells. Anemia can cause fatigue, weakness, paleness, and shortness of breath.

▸ **Esophagitis**: Chronic gastritis can cause acid reflux, which means stomach acids are regurgitated into the esophagus, the tube connecting the mouth to the stomach. Chronic acid reflux can irritate and damage the esophagus's lining, causing esophagitis. Esophagitis can cause symptoms such as heartburn, chest pain, difficulty swallowing, and burning.

▸ **Pyloric stenosis**: Chronic gastritis can sometimes narrow the opening between the stomach and small intestine, causing pyloric stenosis. This can make it difficult for food to pass from the stomach into the small intestine, leading to nausea, vomiting, and weight loss.

▸ **Stomach cancer**: Although rare, untreated or poorly controlled, chronic gastritis may slightly increase the risk of developing stomach cancer. Chronic H. pylori infection, in particular, has been associated with an increased risk of gastric cancer. It is important to note that most people with gastritis will not develop cancer, but regular medical follow-up and proper treatment of gastritis are essential to minimize the risk.

▸ **Gastrointestinal bleeding**: Chronic gastritis can increase the risk of bleeding in the gastrointestinal tract. This can occur when blood vessels in the stomach lining become damaged or eroded, resulting in bleeding. Symptoms of gastrointestinal bleeding may include vomiting blood, black, tarry stools (called melena), weakness, and dizziness. Gastrointestinal bleeding can be a severe complication that requires immediate medical attention.

▸ **Malnutrition**: Chronic inflammation of the stomach lining can affect the absorption of essential nutrients, leading to malnutrition. If the stomach cannot properly break down and absorb food, the body does not receive the nutrients it needs to function correctly. Malnutrition can lead to various health problems, such as muscle weakness, weight loss, growth problems in children, and nutritional deficiencies.

▸ **Gastric obstruction**: In rare cases, chronic gastritis can cause scar tissue in the stomach, leading to gastric obstruction. This can make it difficult or impossible for food to pass from the stomach to the small intestine. Symptoms of gastric obstruction may include severe abdominal pain, nausea, vomiting and bloating. This is a serious complication that usually requires urgent medical intervention.

▸ **Increased risk of other digestive diseases**: Chronic gastritis may increase the risk of developing other digestive diseases, such as gastroesophageal reflux disease (GERD), inflammatory bowel disease (IBD), and Barrett's disease. These diseases may have symptoms similar to gastritis but require different treatment approaches.

‣ **Impact on quality of life**: Chronic gastritis can significantly affect a person's quality of life. Persistent symptoms, such as abdominal pain, nausea and heartburn, can be debilitating and make it difficult to perform routine daily activities. In addition, treatment and management of chronic gastritis may require dietary changes, long-term medications and regular medical follow-up, which can affect a person's routine and comfort.

It is important to note that not everyone with gastritis will develop long-term complications. The severity and likelihood of such complications can vary based on the underlying cause of gastritis, the response to treatment, and other individual factors. However, with the proper knowledge and resources, it is possible to take control of the condition, prevent or effectively manage complications, and strive for an improved quality of life. Remember, it's never too late to prioritize your health and feel your best!

Symptom Reduction and Prevention

Below are some practical recommendations to help alleviate gastritis symptoms and/or prevent its onset, promoting improved digestive health and overall well-being:

‣ **Avoid triggers**: Identifying and avoiding factors that trigger or worsen gastritis symptoms is crucial. Some of these factors may include excessive alcohol consumption, smoking, long-term use of NSAIDs such as ibuprofen or aspirin, and chronic stress. Avoiding or limiting exposure to these factors can help reduce inflammation and damage to the gastric mucosa.

‣ **Healthy diet**: Adopting a balanced and nutritious diet is essential for preventing and managing gastritis. Fiber-rich foods, such as fruits, vegetables, and whole grains, are recommended to help reduce inflammation and promote digestive health. It is also essential to limit the consumption of foods that can irritate the stomach, such as spicy, fatty, fried, and acidic foods, as they can aggravate gastritis symptoms.

‣ **Avoid prolonged fasting**: Regular meal times and avoiding prolonged fasting can help prevent gastritis. Prolonged fasting increases the production of hydrochloric acid in the stomach, damaging the gastric mucosa. Small, frequent meals are recommended instead of large, spaced meals.

▸ **Reduce stress**: Chronic stress can trigger or worsen gastritis symptoms. Stress management techniques like meditation, deep breathing, regular exercise, and relaxing quality time can reduce inflammation and improve overall gastric health.

▸ **Treatment of infections**: Proper treatment of gastritis caused by Helicobacter pylori infection is critical to reducing symptoms and preventing complications. This usually involves a physician-supervised combination of antibiotics and medications to reduce stomach acid production.

▸ **Proper use of medications**: If medications such as NSAIDs are necessary, follow the doctor's recommendations and use the lowest dose and shortest duration possible. In addition, it is advisable to take these medications with food to reduce their impact on the stomach.

▸ **Avoid alcohol and tobacco use**: Both excessive alcohol consumption and smoking can aggravate gastritis symptoms and increase the risk of developing complications. Reducing or altogether avoiding alcohol consumption and quitting smoking can have a positive impact on gastric health.

▸ **Avoid irritating foods**: In addition to spicy, fatty, and acidic foods, other foods can irritate the gastric lining and worsen gastritis symptoms. Examples include coffee, tea, carbonated soft drinks, chocolate and processed foods. Each individual may have different food sensitivities, so it is essential to pay attention to foods that trigger or worsen symptoms and avoid them as much as possible.

▸ **Consume anti-inflammatory foods**: Some foods have anti-inflammatory properties and help reduce inflammation in the gastric mucosa. These foods include ginger, turmeric, garlic, fish rich in omega-3 fatty acids (such as salmon and sardines), berries, green leafy vegetables, and probiotic-rich foods such as yogurt and sauerkraut. Incorporating these foods into the diet can be beneficial in relieving symptoms and promoting healing of the gastric lining.

▸ **Manage emotional stress**: In addition to the stress management techniques mentioned above, addressing emotional stress is essential as a comprehensive approach to reducing gastritis symptoms. This may include seeking emotional support, practicing relaxing activities such as yoga or cognitive behavioral therapy, and finding healthy ways to cope with negative emotions. Chronic emotional stress can affect the health of the digestive system and worsen gastritis symptoms.

▸ **Maintain a healthy weight**: Excess weight and obesity have been associated with an increased risk of developing gastritis and other gastrointestinal disorders. Maintaining a healthy weight through a balanced diet and regular exercise can help reduce inflammation and improve overall gastric health.

▸ **Avoid excessive use of over-the-counter analgesics**: In addition to NSAIDs, excessive use of over-the-counter painkillers, such as acetaminophen, may contribute to gastric mucosal irritation and inflammation. It is important to follow treatment recommendations regarding dosage and duration and to consult a physician if these medications need to be used regularly.

▸ **Regular medical check-ups**: Regular medical check-ups are essential, especially if you have a history of gastritis or recurrent symptoms. A medical specialist can evaluate your gastric health, perform diagnostic tests, monitor your response to treatment, and provide personalized recommendations for gastritis care and prevention.

▸ **Avoid excessive consumption of antacids**: While antacids may temporarily relieve gastritis symptoms, excessive use can have counterproductive effects. They can interfere with the absorption of certain nutrients and alter the acid-base balance in the stomach. It is crucial to use antacids only when necessary and under the supervision of a physician.

▸ **Avoid physical stress on the stomach**: Physical stress, such as heavy lifting or high-impact exercise after eating, can increase pressure and cause acid reflux. It is advisable to avoid strenuous activities immediately after meals and give the stomach time to digest food properly.

‣ **Control other health conditions**: Some health conditions, such as gastroesophageal reflux disease (GERD) and celiac disease, can increase the risk of developing gastritis. Properly managing and treating these conditions can help prevent gastritis and decrease symptoms.

‣ **Avoid excessive caffeine intake**: Excessive caffeine intake, whether through coffee, tea, or energy drinks, can increase stomach acid production and worsen gastritis symptoms. Limiting caffeine intake or opting for decaffeinated alternatives may reduce gastric irritation.

‣ **Maintain good food hygiene**: Eating contaminated food or mishandling food can lead to gastrointestinal tract infections, which can cause gastritis. Good food hygiene practices include washing hands before handling food, cooking food to a safe temperature, and ensuring that food is fresh and well-stored.

‣ **Avoid oxidative stress**: Oxidative stress can contribute to inflammation and damage the gastric lining. Eating a diet rich in antioxidants, such as fruits and vegetables, and avoiding excessive consumption of processed foods and saturated fats may help reduce oxidative stress and promote gastric health.

Diagnostic Medical Tests

The following provides detailed information about the medical tests commonly used to diagnose various types of gastritis.

‣ **Upper endoscopy**: Endoscopy is a test commonly used to diagnose gastritis. A thin, flexible tube with a camera on the end (endoscope) is inserted through the mouth into the stomach. It allows the physician to visualize the stomach lining directly and take tissue samples for further analysis (biopsy). Endoscopy can also reveal signs of inflammation, ulcers, or bacterial infections, such as Helicobacter pylori.

- **Blood tests**: Blood tests may be performed to detect the presence of Helicobacter pylori bacteria or to evaluate the levels of specific inflammatory markers in the body. The results of these tests can help determine if the gastritis is related to a bacterial infection or if there are signs of inflammation in the body.

- **Urease test**: This test is performed during endoscopy. A tissue sample is taken from the stomach lining and placed in a urea culture medium. If Helicobacter pylori bacteria are present, they will produce an enzyme called urease, which breaks down urea and produces carbon dioxide. The release of carbon dioxide is detected, confirming the presence of the bacteria.

- **Barium X-ray**: In this test, a barium solution, which coats the lining of the stomach and intestines, is swallowed, and X-rays are taken. This allows the physician to detect any abnormalities in the stomach, such as ulcers or inflammation. However, this test is less commonly used than endoscopy, as it cannot provide as precise details as direct visualization by endoscopy.

- **Breath tests**: These tests are explicitly used to detect the presence of Helicobacter pylori bacteria. The person is asked to swallow a substance containing urea labeled with carbon-13 or carbon-14. If the bacteria are present in the stomach, they will break down the urea and release carbon dioxide, which will be detected in the person's breath.

- **Laboratory tests**: Blood tests may also include evaluating hemoglobin levels and blood cells, which can help identify possible anemia caused by chronic gastritis. In addition, tests may be performed to detect nutritional deficiencies, such as a lack of vitamin B12 resulting from malabsorption due to chronic gastritis.

- **Esophageal pH test**: This test evaluates the acidity of the esophagus to determine if acid reflux is present. During the procedure, a small, thin tube is placed through the nose or mouth into the esophagus. The tube measures the level of acidity in the esophagus over 24 hours. Frequent acid reflux can irritate the stomach lining and contribute to gastritis.

‣ **Gastric emptying test**: This test evaluates the rate at which the stomach empties. A food or drink containing a small amount of radioactive material is swallowed. Images are then taken at regular intervals to track the movement of the material through the stomach and intestines. This test can help identify if there is a delay in gastric emptying, which may contribute to gastritis.

‣ **Food allergy testing**: In some cases, gastritis may be triggered by food allergies or intolerances. Allergy testing, such as skin or blood testing, can be performed to identify food allergens contributing to gastritis symptoms.

‣ **Lactulose breath test**: This test evaluates the presence and overgrowth of bacteria in the small intestine, which can contribute to gastritis. The person is asked to drink lactulose and take breath samples regularly. Bacteria in the small intestine can ferment lactulose and produce gas, which can be detected in the person's breath.

It is important to note that not all of these tests are necessary to diagnose gastritis. The choice of the most appropriate tests will be based on the physician's judgment, considering your symptoms, medical history, and findings from the physical examination.

Warning Signs

The presence of certain symptoms may suggest a serious digestive disorder. If you notice any of the following signs, it is essential to seek immediate medical attention.

‣ Complete loss of appetite.
‣ Fever or fever for no apparent reason lasting several days.
‣ Vague discomfort in the abdomen, just above the navel, lasting more than one week.
‣ A feeling of fullness in the upper abdomen after eating a little.
‣ Unintentional weight loss without dieting.

- Nausea and vomiting, especially vomiting of solid foods shortly after eating.
- Swelling or accumulation of fluid in the abdomen.
- Pain or sensation of food getting "stuck" in the throat when eating.
- Chronic heartburn or indigestion.
- Persistent vomiting, with or without blood.
- Black stools.
- Anemia.
- Palpation of a lump or mass in the area of the pit of the stomach (epigastrium).
- Jaundice, i.e., yellowing of the skin and whites of the eyes.
- Family history of gastrointestinal cancer.

The presence of these symptoms does not necessarily mean a condition such as cancer. However, seeking prompt medical attention is crucial to rule out any serious issues and to obtain an accurate diagnosis, ensuring the necessary treatment is received.

FREQUENTLY ASKED QUESTIONS

Navigating the intricate world of health can feel overwhelming, especially when faced with a diagnosis that affects both physical and emotional well-being. In such moments, many questions naturally arise: What does this mean for me? What options are available? How will my daily life change? Uncertainty and concern are common. Here, you'll discover practical and direct insights to help you make confident, informed choices.

This chapter was created to offer support and provide clear, straightforward tools to guide you through this journey. In today's era of abundant information, distinguishing reliable knowledge from content that might cause confusion is vital. With this in mind, I've compiled evidence-based guidance to help you navigate uncertainty with greater clarity.

The format of this resource prioritizes accessibility, addressing common concerns faced by individuals and families alike. Each explanation is concise, clear, and aimed at empowering you to make decisions that align with your overall well-being.

While the material here is designed to assist, it is not a substitute for personalized advice from healthcare professionals. Consulting your doctor for guidance tailored to your specific needs remains essential, especially to address challenges unique to your situation.

Through these pages, my goal is to foster calm, confidence, and reassurance so that you can approach your circumstances with strength and resolve. I hope this resource inspires you and provides the valuable tools necessary to manage your health effectively and confidently.

124 FAQs about Gastritis

1. What are the most common causes of gastritis?

The most common causes of gastritis include infection by Helicobacter pylori bacteria, prolonged use of non-steroidal anti-inflammatory drugs (NSAIDs), excessive alcohol consumption, chronic stress and autoimmune diseases.

2. What are the symptoms of gastritis?

Gastritis symptoms may include pain or discomfort in the upper abdomen, nausea, vomiting, a feeling of fullness after eating, loss of appetite, and, in some cases, gastrointestinal bleeding.

3. What tests are used to diagnose gastritis?

Gastritis is diagnosed through medical history and various tests, such as endoscopy, biopsy of the stomach lining, blood tests, breath tests for Helicobacter pylori, and stool analysis.

4. Are there home tests to diagnose gastritis?

Currently, there are no reliable home tests to diagnose gastritis. A proper medical evaluation, which may include endoscopies and laboratory tests, is required.

5. What medical treatments are available for gastritis?

Treatment for gastritis depends on its cause. It may include antibiotics to treat Helicobacter pylori infection, medications to reduce stomach acid production, such as proton pump inhibitors or H2 blockers, and diet and lifestyle changes to avoid stomach irritants.

6. Can gastritis develop into a more serious condition?

If not adequately treated, gastritis can lead to complications such as gastric ulcers, bleeding of the stomach lining, and an increased risk of stomach cancer in chronic cases or associated with prolonged Helicobacter pylori infections.

7. What foods should I avoid if I have gastritis?

It is advisable to avoid foods that may irritate the stomach, such as spicy, acidic, fried foods, and alcoholic or caffeinated beverages. The corresponding chapter will discuss these in detail.

8. Can I eat spicy foods or spices if I have gastritis?
Spicy foods and spices can irritate the stomach and aggravate gastritis symptoms in some people. If they cause discomfort, it is best to avoid or consume them in moderation.

9. Are there foods that can help cure gastritis?
Yes, some foods can help cure gastritis. These include natural yogurt, which contains probiotics, and green leafy vegetables, which are rich in fiber and help maintain a healthy digestive system and alleviate some symptoms of gastritis. We will see this in the corresponding chapter. b

10. Can gastritis be caused by an unbalanced diet?
A diet high in irritating foods, such as spicy, fatty, or processed foods, may contribute to developing gastritis or worsen its symptoms.

11. Is gastritis contagious?
Gastritis itself is not contagious, but Helicobacter pylori infection, one of the most common causes of gastritis, can be transmitted from person to person through direct contact with saliva, vomit, or feces, or by consuming contaminated food and water.

12. Can I prevent gastritis?
To prevent gastritis, it is essential to maintain a healthy diet, limit the use of NSAIDs, moderate alcohol consumption, avoid smoking, and manage stress. Following proper hygiene practices to prevent Helicobacter pylori infections is also important.

13. Can gastritis be caused by stress?
Yes, stress can contribute to the development of gastritis by increasing stomach acid production and affecting the functioning of the digestive system.

14. Can emotional stress worsen gastritis?
Yes, emotional stress can increase stomach acid production and worsen gastritis symptoms. Stress management techniques can help relieve symptoms.

15. Can physical stress trigger gastritis?

Physical stress, such as severe illness or surgery, can cause acute gastritis by increasing stomach acid production or reducing blood flow to the stomach.

16. Is gastritis a chronic condition?

Gastritis can be acute or chronic. Acute gastritis appears suddenly and may be caused by irritants such as alcohol or NSAIDs. Chronic gastritis develops gradually and may be caused mainly by persistent Helicobacter pylori infections or autoimmune diseases.

17. Does gastritis affect people of all ages?

Yes, gastritis can affect people of any age, although certain risk factors, such as NSAID use, Helicobacter pylori infection and alcohol consumption, may be more common in adults.

18. Do I need to modify my lifestyle if I have gastritis?

Yes, lifestyle changes can help manage and prevent gastritis. These may include adopting a healthy diet, avoiding alcohol and tobacco use, managing stress, and avoiding excessive use of NSAIDs.

19. Can I drink coffee if I have gastritis?

Coffee, especially caffeinated coffee, can irritate the stomach and aggravate gastritis symptoms. If symptoms occur, it is recommended to limit or avoid coffee consumption.

20. Is decaffeinated coffee better for gastritis?

Decaffeinated coffee can be less irritating than regular coffee, but it can still stimulate acid production in the stomach. It is advisable to observe individual tolerance.

21. Can gastritis cause weight loss?

Yes, gastritis can lead to unintentional weight loss due to decreased appetite, malabsorption of nutrients, and digestive discomfort, making it difficult to eat correctly.

22. Can gastritis cause changes in appetite?

Yes, gastritis can cause a decreased appetite due to pain and discomfort when eating, although some people may experience an increased appetite if eating relieves the pain.

23. Are there natural remedies to alleviate the symptoms?

Some natural remedies, such as chamomile tea, ginger and aloe vera, help relieve gastritis symptoms. We will discuss this in detail in the corresponding chapter.

24. How long does it take for gastritis to heal?

Recovery time for gastritis varies depending on its cause and severity. With appropriate treatment, acute gastritis may resolve in a few days to weeks, while chronic gastritis may require more prolonged treatment and ongoing lifestyle management.

25. Is gastritis the same as an ulcer?

No, gastritis and ulcers are different conditions. Gastritis is inflammation of the stomach lining, while an ulcer is an open sore in the stomach lining or small intestine. However, gastritis can increase the risk of developing ulcers.

26. Is physical exercise recommended?

Moderate exercise benefits digestion, health and overall well-being, but avoiding activities that worsen gastritis symptoms, such as high-intensity exercise immediately after eating, is essential. Listen to your body and avoid intense exercise if it causes stomach discomfort.

27. Can I continue exercising if I have gastritis?

Yes, you can usually continue to exercise if you have gastritis. However, listening to your body and avoiding activities that aggravate your symptoms is essential. Moderate exercise can even help reduce stress, which is a factor that often worsens gastritis.

28. Can gastritis affect sleep?

Yes, gastritis symptoms, such as pain, nausea and abdominal discomfort, can interfere with sleep. Maintaining a proper diet and avoiding heavy meals and irritating drinks before bedtime can help improve insomnia or interrupted sleep.

29. Is it safe to use antacids for gastritis in the long term?

Antacids may temporarily relieve gastritis by neutralizing stomach acid, but do not address the underlying cause. A physician should supervise their prolonged use, as they may affect nutrient absorption and have other side effects.

30. Does the consumption of probiotics help?
Probiotics can help restore the healthy balance of the intestinal microbiota and improve digestive health, primarily if the gastritis is related to Helicobacter pylori infection.

31. Can gastritis cause bad breath?
Yes, gastritis can contribute to bad breath, mainly if associated with a Helicobacter pylori infection. This infection can affect the bacterial balance in the mouth and stomach.

32. Can I drink milk if I have gastritis?
Milk may temporarily relieve the stomach lining, but it may also stimulate acid production, which could aggravate symptoms in the long term. Therefore, it is advisable to consult with a healthcare professional to determine whether including milk in your case is appropriate.

33. What role does the immune system play in gastritis?
In some cases, gastritis is caused by an autoimmune response in which the immune system attacks the stomach lining cells, causing chronic inflammation. This form of gastritis is known as autoimmune gastritis.

34. Can gastritis cause fever?
Although fever is not a common symptom of gastritis, in cases where gastritis is caused by an infection (such as Helicobacter pylori infection), there may be an associated fever.

35. Is fasting recommended for gastritis?
Prolonged fasting is not usually recommended for gastritis, as an empty stomach can increase acid production and aggravate symptoms. It is better to opt for small, frequent meals.

36. Does "intermittent fasting" affect gastritis?
Intermittent fasting has variable or mixed effects on gastritis. For some people, it may improve symptoms by resting the digestive system; for others, it may increase acidity and irritation, worsening symptoms.

37. Can gastritis cause problems in other parts of the digestive system?
If not treated, gastritis can develop into more severe problems, such as ulcers, affecting other parts of the digestive system, such as the duodenum.

38. Can gastritis cause acid reflux?
Yes, gastritis can be associated with acid reflux. Stomach inflammation can affect the function of the lower esophageal sphincter, allowing stomach acid to back up into the esophagus.

39. Is acid reflux related to gastritis?
Acid reflux and gastritis are different conditions, but they can co-occur. Acid reflux can increase the symptoms of gastritis and vice versa.

40. Can I take vitamin supplements if I have gastritis?
Some vitamin supplements can irritate the stomach, especially if taken on an empty stomach. It is best to consult a health professional about which vitamin supplements are suitable if you have gastritis.

41. Is the use of digestive enzyme supplements recommended for gastritis?
Digestive enzymes help some people improve digestion and reduce the burden on the stomach.

42. Is it safe to take omega-3 supplements?
Omega-3s have anti-inflammatory properties that can be beneficial. However, it is essential to consult a health professional, as some people may experience stomach upset.

43. Is it safe to take vitamin C supplements with gastritis?
Vitamin C can be beneficial, but large amounts can irritate the stomach. It is better to consume it with food and consult a specialist.

44. Is it safe for people with gastritis to take calcium supplements?
Calcium is essential, but some forms of supplements can cause stomach upset. It is best to opt for more easily absorbable forms

and consult a professional.

45. Is using iron supplements safe?
Iron supplements can be irritating to the stomach. To minimize the risk of irritation, they should be taken with food and under medical supervision.

46. Does gastritis affect the absorption of nutrients?
Chronic gastritis, mainly associated with gastric atrophy, can affect the absorption of certain nutrients, such as iron and vitamin B12, leading to nutritional deficiencies.

47. Can gastritis cause anemia?
Yes, chronic gastritis, mainly caused by atrophy of the stomach lining, can lead to malabsorption of essential nutrients such as iron and vitamin B12, which can cause anemia.

48. Can gastritis cause fatigue?
Yes, gastritis can lead to fatigue and weakness due to malabsorption of nutrients, continuous pain, anemia, sleep disorders, or lack of appetite.

49. Can gastritis cause drug absorption problems?
Stomach inflammation can affect the absorption of certain medications, so it is essential to inform the doctor about gastritis so that treatments can be adjusted if necessary.

50. Can gastritis cause dizziness?
Although dizziness is not a direct symptom of gastritis, malabsorption of nutrients and dehydration associated with digestive problems may contribute to the feeling of dizziness.

51. Can gastritis affect the skin?
Malabsorption of nutrients due to gastritis can affect the skin's health, sometimes causing dryness, paleness, or rashes.

52. Does chocolate consumption affect gastritis?
Chocolate may increase stomach acid production and relax the lower esophageal sphincter, which can worsen gastritis symptoms in some people. If symptoms occur, consuming chocolate in moderation or avoiding it is advisable.

53. Can gastritis be treated with surgery?
Surgery is not a standard treatment for gastritis. However, in very severe cases where there are complications such as perforated ulcers, surgical treatment may be necessary.

54. What role do genetics play in gastritis?
While genetics may influence susceptibility to certain diseases, gastritis is more often related to environmental factors, infections and lifestyle habits.

55. Can gastritis be hereditary?
Although gastritis is not usually hereditary, some conditions that predispose to gastritis, such as certain autoimmune diseases, may have a genetic component.

56. Is green tea good for gastritis?
Green tea contains antioxidants that can benefit digestive health. However, it also contains caffeine, which can irritate the stomach in some people. Therefore, it is best to consume it in moderation, observe how your body reacts, or opt for decaffeinated varieties.

57. Can gastritis cause changes in bowel habits?
Gastritis can affect digestion, which may result in changes in bowel habits, such as diarrhea or constipation, although these are not significant symptoms.

58. What role does the intestinal microbiota play?
A healthy gut microbiota can help protect the stomach lining and reduce inflammation, while an imbalance can contribute to digestive problems, including gastritis.

59. How does tobacco affect gastritis?
Smoking can increase stomach acid production and weaken the stomach's protective barrier, worsening the symptoms of gastritis and making it more difficult to heal.

60. Does gastritis always require medical treatment?
Although mild cases of gastritis may resolve with diet and lifestyle changes, it is advisable to seek medical advice to determine the underlying cause and receive treatment,

especially if symptoms persist.

61. Do carbonated soft drinks affect gastritis?
Carbonated beverages can increase acid production and cause bloating, worsening gastritis symptoms.

62. Is ginger beneficial for gastritis?
Ginger has anti-inflammatory properties and helps relieve nausea and soothe the stomach. However, some people may find it irritating, so it is essential to try it in small amounts.

63. Can gastritis cause back pain?
Although uncommon, severe stomach pain associated with gastritis may radiate to the back. It is essential to consult a physician to rule out other possible causes of back pain.

64. Can gastritis be caused by medications?
Yes, certain medications, especially non-steroidal anti-inflammatory drugs (NSAIDs) such as ibuprofen and aspirin, can irritate the stomach lining and cause gastritis.

65. Is garlic harmful for gastritis?
Garlic has antimicrobial and anti-inflammatory properties, but it can irritate the stomach of people with gastritis. It is best to consume it in small amounts to see how it affects symptoms.

66. How does alcohol affect gastritis?
Alcohol consumption can irritate and erode the stomach lining, worsening the symptoms of gastritis and making it more difficult to heal.

67. Is vinegar beneficial for gastritis?
Although some claim that vinegar helps balance the stomach's pH, it can irritate the gastric lining and is not generally recommended for gastritis.

68. Can gastritis be a risk factor for other diseases?
Yes, if left untreated, chronic gastritis can increase the risk of developing stomach ulcers, iron deficiency anemia, and, in some cases, stomach cancer.

69. Can chronic gastritis lead to stomach cancer?
Chronic gastritis, mainly when caused by Helicobacter pylori, can increase the risk of developing stomach cancer in the long term. It is crucial to treat the infection properly to reduce this risk.

70. Can gastritis cause abdominal bloating?
Yes, gastritis can cause bloating and fullness due to inflammation of the stomach lining and excessive gas production.

71. Can gastritis cause gas?
Yes, gastritis can cause a buildup of gas in the stomach, resulting in belching or flatulence.

72. Are small, frequent meals recommended for gastritis?
Yes, eating small, frequent meals helps reduce the burden on the stomach and minimizes gastritis symptoms.

73. Is chamomile tea good for gastritis?
Chamomile is known for its soothing and anti-inflammatory properties and helps relieve some symptoms of gastritis, such as pain and nausea.

74. How does aging affect gastritis?
As we age, the stomach lining can become thinner and more susceptible to irritation, increasing the risk of developing gastritis.

75. Can strong emotions aggravate gastritis?
Strong emotions such as anxiety or stress do not cause gastritis directly, but may exacerbate symptoms due to increased stomach acid production.

76. Can gastritis cause changes in bowel movements?
Although gastritis primarily affects the stomach, associated digestive problems, such as diarrhea or constipation, can lead to changes in bowel movements.

77. Can gastritis cause changes in the stool?
Yes, gastritis can lead to changes in the stool, such as darker

stools, if there is bleeding in the stomach.

78. Is aloe vera beneficial for gastritis?
Aloe vera is known for its anti-inflammatory properties and helps soothe the stomach lining. Choosing products that do not contain aloin is important, but it can be irritating. It is essential to consult a healthcare professional before using it as a treatment, as it may have adverse effects on some people or interact with some drugs. You will find more information in the chapter "Medicinal Plants".

79. Can acid-reducing medications cause side effects?
Yes, proton pump inhibitors (PPIs) and other acid-reducing drugs can have side effects, such as diarrhea, constipation, or nutrient deficiency if used long-term. Check with your doctor or pharmacist.

80. Can yoga and meditation help with gastritis?
Practices such as yoga and meditation help reduce stress, which indirectly helps alleviate gastritis symptoms by decreasing stomach acid production and improving overall well-being.

81. Can food allergies cause gastritis?
Although food allergies are not a common cause of gastritis, they can cause digestive symptoms that could be mistaken for gastritis.

82. How does the menstrual cycle influence gastritis?
Some women may experience a worsening of gastritis symptoms during the menstrual cycle due to hormonal changes that affect stomach acid production and gastro-intestinal sensitivity.

83. How does dehydration affect gastritis?
Dehydration can worsen gastritis by concentrating acids in the stomach and making digestion difficult, so it is crucial to maintain good hydration.

84. Is the consumption of water with lemon* good?
Although lemon* is acidic, some people find that lemon water in small amounts helps with digestion. However, it can irritate

the stomach in others, so it is essential to try it cautiously and assess personal tolerance. (*See the "Foods That Transform" chapter, "Lemon and Gastritis: Myth or Remedy?" section for more information).

85. What is the role of hydrochloric acid in gastritis?
Hydrochloric acid is essential for digestion, but excess can damage the stomach lining and contribute to gastritis.

86. Can gastritis cause vomiting?
Yes, inflammation and irritation of the stomach can cause nausea and vomiting in people with gastritis.

87. Is it possible to have gastritis without apparent symptoms?
Yes, some people may have mild gastritis, inflammation present, but without obvious symptoms.

88. How does gastritis affect children?
Children may experience symptoms similar to adults, such as abdominal pain and nausea. Causes in children may include infections, use of medications, and stress.

89. Is pure bee honey good for gastritis?
Pure bee honey has beneficial antibacterial, anti-inflammatory, antioxidant, and antimicrobial properties. However, it is essential to consume it in moderation and observe how your body reacts.

90. What is the relationship between Helicobacter pylori and gastritis?
Helicobacter pylori is a bacterium that can infect the stomach. It is one of the most common causes of chronic gastritis, which can lead to inflammation of the stomach lining.

91. Is turmeric recommended for gastritis?
Turmeric has anti-inflammatory and antioxidant properties and may be beneficial in reducing inflammation. However, it should be used cautiously, as it may irritate the stomach in some people.

92. Is the consumption of clear soups beneficial?
Clear soups are easy to digest and help maintain hydration, making them a good choice for individuals with gastritis.

93. Is chicken soup good for gastritis?
Chicken soup is usually gentle on the stomach and, if it does not contain strong spices or irritating ingredients, can be a good choice for people with gastritis.

94. How does body posture influence gastritis?
Maintaining good posture and avoiding lying down immediately after eating helps reduce acid reflux, which can exacerbate gastritis symptoms.

95. Does drinking hot water help with gastritis?
Drinking hot water can help soothe the stomach by improving digestion and relieving stomach spasms, but it should not be too hot to avoid irritation.

96. Can gastritis cause depression or anxiety?
Chronic gastritis and persistent pain can affect quality of life and contribute to mental health problems such as depression or anxiety.

97. Is yogurt recommended for people with gastritis?
Yogurt, specifically those that contain probiotics, can often help balance intestinal flora. However, it is essential to choose low-fat varieties with no added sugars.

98. Is the consumption of fiber beneficial for gastritis?
A fiber-rich diet can help improve digestion and prevent irritation of the gastric lining, but it is important to introduce it gradually.

99. Is oat consumption recommended for gastritis?
Oatmeal is a soft food rich in soluble fiber, which can benefit the stomach lining and help reduce acidity.

100. Is coconut oil recommended for gastritis?
Some people use coconut oil for its antimicrobial properties, but its effect varies from person to person. It is best to consume

it in small amounts to see how it affects symptoms.

101. Is coconut water consumption beneficial?
Coconut water is mild and can help maintain hydration without irritating the stomach. It is also a source of electrolytes, making it a good option for people with gastritis.

102. Is the consumption of bananas good for gastritis?
Bananas are gentle on the stomach and can help neutralize acidity, providing mild relief from gastritis symptoms.

103. Is the consumption of bananas recommended?
Bananas are soft, easy to digest, and rich in nutrients, making them suitable for people with gastritis.

104. Can gastritis cause a feeling of rapid satiety?
Yes, stomach lining inflammation can make you feel full quickly, even after eating small amounts of food.

105. Is the consumption of papaya recommended?
Papaya contains papain, an enzyme that facilitates digestion and relieves stomach upset. Thus, it is a good choice for most people with gastritis. However, the effect on gastritis may vary according to individual sensitivity.

106. Is the consumption of white rice recommended?
White rice is easy to digest and gentle on the stomach, making it suitable for people with gastritis.

107. Can gastritis cause chest pain?
Although chest pain is not a typical symptom of gastritis, the associated acid reflux can cause a burning sensation or pain in the chest. It is essential to seek medical attention to rule out heart problems.

108. Can gastritis cause constipation?
Although gastritis is most commonly associated with diarrhea, changes in diet or stress can also cause constipation in some people.

109. Is pumpkin consumption recommended?

Pumpkin is a soft and easy-to-digest food that benefits people with gastritis.

110. Can gastritis cause excessive sweating?
Excessive sweating is not a common symptom of gastritis, but may occur in response to pain or anxiety related to the disease.

111. Can gastritis cause night sweats?
Although not a common symptom, night sweats may occur if the gastritis is related to an infection or causes significant discomfort that affects sleep.

112. Is potato consumption recommended for gastritis?
Potatoes, especially when cooked and without irritating seasonings, are mild and are usually well tolerated by people with gastritis.

113. Can gastritis cause a sore throat?
Although not a direct symptom, acid reflux associated with gastritis can irritate the throat and cause pain.

114. Is the consumption of carrots recommended for gastritis?
Carrots are rich in nutrients and generally gentle on the stomach, which makes them suitable for people with gastritis.

115. Can gastritis cause palpitations?
Palpitations are not a typical symptom of gastritis, but pain or stress related to the disease may contribute to an increased perception of the heartbeat.

116. Is fish consumption recommended for gastritis?
Lean fish, such as white fish, are easy to digest and can be a good source of protein for people with gastritis.

117. Can gastritis cause headaches?
Although not a direct symptom, the stress and discomfort associated with gastritis may contribute to headaches in some people.

118. Can gastritis cause ringing in the ears?

Ringing in the ears is not a typical symptom of gastritis, but stress or anxiety related to the disease may contribute to this symptom.

119. Is the consumption of steamed food beneficial for gastritis?
Steamed foods are soft and easy to digest, making them a good option for people with gastritis.

120. Which medicinal plants are recommended?
Plants such as chamomile, ginger and licorice (in the form of DGL) are commonly used to relieve gastritis symptoms. We will discuss these in the corresponding chapter.

121. Is deglycyrrhizinated licorice safe for gastritis?
DGL is a licorice that does not contain glycyrrhizin, a compound that can raise blood pressure. It may help protect the stomach lining and is considered safe for most people with gastritis.

122. Is peppermint recommended for gastritis?
Peppermint can relieve some stomach discomfort but also relaxes the lower esophageal sphincter, which may worsen reflux in some people. Therefore, it should be used cautiously and tested to see how it works for you.

123. Can I use peppermint oil to relieve stomach pain?
Peppermint oil may help relieve intestinal spasms, but it may aggravate acid reflux. It should be used with caution and under medical supervision.

124. Can fennel relieve the symptoms of gastritis?
Fennel is known for its carminative properties and often helps to relieve bloating and stomach upset.

SUGGESTED PRACTICAL PLAN

In this chapter, you will find a clear, practical, and easy-to-follow plan designed to help you effectively manage and alleviate gastritis. This guide focuses on the most vital aspects of care, offering a straightforward path to progressively restore your health and well-being. Let's dive in and start your journey to recovery!

▸ **Understand the Root Causes**: Start by identifying the root causes of your gastritis and taking steps to eliminate or minimize them. Addressing these underlying factors is a crucial first step in your recovery journey. For more details, refer to the chapter "Gastritis" under the section titled "Causes".

▸ **Consider Nutritional Supplements**: Nutritional supplements can be an excellent addition to your treatment plan, providing extra support to your recovery process. Choose specific supplements mentioned in the relevant chapter or follow a tailored combination of recommendations for optimal results.

▸ **Incorporate Phytotherapy**: Medicinal plants can play a valuable role in your recovery. Explore the chapter "Medicinal Plants" for a carefully curated list of plants and recipes designed to promote healing and support your stomach's health naturally.

▸ **Focus on Your Diet**: Diet is one of the most impactful aspects when managing gastritis. Following the dietary guidelines shared in the chapter "Gastritis" under the section titled "Symptom Reduction and Prevention" is fundamental. Don't miss the chapters "Foods That Transform" and "Juices and Smoothies", where you'll find invaluable insights, over 50 recipes for daily meal plans, and delicious beverages specifically crafted to improve your stomach's health.

‣ **Review Medications**: If any of your current medications appear to trigger or worsen your symptoms, it's crucial to consult with your doctor. They can help revise your treatment protocol or adjust dosages to better align with your healing process.

‣ **Lifestyle**: Your lifestyle choices significantly impact your gastritis symptoms. Practical tips and routines for healthier habits can be found in the section "Symptom Reduction and Prevention."

‣ **Regular exercise**: Staying active is essential. Exercise helps maintain a healthy weight and reduces stress levels, both of which are important in managing gastritis. However, ensure you leave at least three hours between meals and physical activity to avoid digestive discomfort.

‣ **Relaxation techniques**: Practices like yoga, tai chi, and meditation go beyond relaxation–they help release emotional tension and stress, which can positively impact your recovery from gastritis.

Address Related Conditions
If you are managing additional issues like acid reflux, SIBO, or constipation alongside gastritis, consider exploring the remedies presented in my other books:

- ‣ **ACID REFLUX**. Foods, Supplements and Medicinal Plants
- ‣ **CONSTIPATION**. Foods, Supplements and Medicinal Plants
- ‣ **HEMORRHOIDS**. Food, Supplements and Medicinal Plants
- ‣ **SIBO**. Foods, Supplements and Medicinal Plants

This plan combines scientifically proven principles with a user-friendly approach, empowering you to take proactive steps in improving your quality of life and finding lasting relief from gastritis. Remember, you are not alone in this journey–stay hopeful, take things one step at a time, and believe in your capacity to heal. Your path to wellness starts here!

NUTRITIONAL SUPPLEMENTS

Nutritional supplements have become a valuable ally in the pursuit of better health and an enhanced quality of life. These options–available in various user-friendly formats such as tablets, capsules, powders, or easily consumable liquids–are purposefully designed to complement your daily nutrition by delivering essential nutrients that can be challenging to obtain through regular meals alone. Packed with powerful components like vitamins, minerals, amino acids, antioxidants, and other bioactive compounds, these supplements are expertly formulated in precise proportions to meet the unique needs of every individual–even when the demands are high. Whether you're navigating restrictive diets, facing nutritional gaps, or coping with increased physical or mental demands, supplements can provide the extra support your body needs.

Beyond simply filling in nutritional gaps, supplements offer an array of tailored benefits to suit diverse lifestyles and health challenges. They can help boost energy, improve physical performance, support those managing fast-paced lives, and provide practical solutions for staying balanced and resilient. Their significance often becomes even more apparent during times of illness, specific health conditions, or chronic issues. In these situations, supplements do more than complement a diet– they can actively help restore altered functions, ease symptoms, and assist in more complex recovery processes. They serve as companions in the pursuit of health, helping you sustain and rebuild your vitality.

Effectively integrating supplements into your routine requires thoughtful use grounded in science and, when needed, professional guidance. By understanding their benefits and approaching them with care, supplements can evolve into powerful tools for improving your overall well-being in a sustainable and meaningful way. Remember–every step you take toward caring for your body is a step closer to feeling stronger, more energized, and more capable of facing life's challenges with confidence. Take that step today. Your path to better health begins with small but impactful choices!

Essential Precautions

Understanding the risks associated with supplements is vital, as they can sometimes cause side effects, have contraindications, or interact with medications. It's important to thoroughly review the potential adverse effects detailed at the end of this chapter. Take a moment to assess your overall health and avoid any supplements that could conflict with the medications you're currently taking or exacerbate existing medical conditions. Prioritizing this step ensures a safer and more effective approach to improving your well-being.

Nutritional Supplements and Gastritis

When it comes to gastritis, nutritional supplements can be an invaluable tool for supporting gastric health. These supplements play a key role in correcting nutritional deficiencies, promoting the repair of the gastric mucosa, and reducing inflammation, all of which contribute significantly to symptom relief.

In this chapter, you'll discover the most effective and widely recognized nutritional supplements for managing gastritis. To make it easier for you, we've organized them alphabetically so you can find them quickly. You can choose to use one or two supplements individually, or explore the **"Strategic Supplement Combinations"** recommended in the next section to maximize their benefits.

Chamomile

Chamomile is a medicinal herb known for its soothing properties and its traditional use in treating various digestive disorders. It has long been used as a natural remedy to relieve gastrointestinal symptoms.

Benefits:
- Anti-inflammatory action: It contains anti-inflammatory

compounds that help reduce inflammation in the stomach lining.

‣ Relief of digestive symptoms: It has traditionally been used to relieve symptoms such as heartburn, indigestion, cramps and gastrointestinal discomfort that may be present in gastritis.

‣ Soothing effect: It has calming properties and helps reduce discomfort and irritation in the stomach.

Recommended dosage:
The recommended dose ranges from 300 to 1300 mg per day, depending on the concentration of the product.

Posology:
It is recommended to take it once or twice a day. It promotes relaxation and sleep if taken at night before going to bed. According to personal preference, it can be taken with or without food.

Average action time:
The time of onset of action may vary, but the effect usually appears after a few days to a few weeks of continuous use.

Maximum recommended time of continuous use:
There is no established maximum time. If it is planned to be used consecutively for more than six months, follow the manufacturer's instructions or consult a specialist.

Curcumin

Curcumin, an active compound present in turmeric, has gained popularity due to its benefits for gastritis.

Benefits:
‣ Anti-inflammatory action: Curcumin has been shown to have anti-inflammatory properties that help reduce inflammation in the stomach lining caused by gastritis.

‣ Stomach lining protection: This helps strengthen the

protective barrier of the stomach lining, which can prevent damage and irritation caused by gastritis.

‣ Antioxidant properties: It is known for its potent antioxidant properties, which help fight oxidative stress and protect the cells of the stomach lining against free radical damage.

Recommended dosage:
The recommended dose ranges from 300 mg to 1500 mg per day.

Posology:
Taking it once or twice a day, with meals, is recommended to improve its absorption.

Average action time:
The average action time may vary, but it usually shows an effect within a few weeks of continuous use.

Maximum recommended time of continuous use:
There is no defined maximum time for continuous use. However, it is advisable to consult a specialist if you plan to use it for more than six months in a row, especially in high doses.

Ginger

Ginger is a root widely used in cooking and traditional medicine due to its medicinal properties. Ginger has been researched for its potential to relieve gastrointestinal symptoms and promote overall digestive health.

Benefits:
‣ Anti-inflammatory properties: It contains compounds with anti-inflammatory properties, which help reduce inflammation in the stomach lining associated with gastritis.

‣ Relief of digestive symptoms: Ginger has traditionally been used to relieve symptoms of stomach discomfort, such as nausea, vomiting and fullness, which may be present in gastritis.

‣ Stomach lining protection: Ginger's compounds help strengthen the stomach's protective barrier, protecting the lining from damage.

Recommended dosage:
The recommended dose ranges from 500 to 2000 mg per day, depending on the concentration of the product.

Posology:
It would be best to take it once or twice a day, preferably in the morning and/or evening. You can take it with or without food, but some people prefer to take it with meals to avoid possible stomach upset.

Average action time:
The time of onset of action may vary, but the effect usually appears after a few days to a few weeks of continuous use.

Maximum recommended time of continuous use:
There is no established maximum time for continuous use. If use is planned for more than six months, it is recommended to follow the manufacturer's instructions or consult a specialist.

Glutamine

Glutamine is an amino acid considered essential for the health and proper functioning of the intestinal lining.

Benefits:
‣ Repair and maintenance of the intestinal lining: Glutamine may play an essential role in repairing and maintaining the intestinal lining, which is beneficial for stomach health and treating gastritis.

‣ Strengthening the immune system: Glutamine helps strengthen the immune system and promotes proper bowel function, reducing inflammation and improving the immune response in gastritis.

‣ Digestive health support: Contributes to the overall health of the digestive system, including the stomach, by helping to maintain the integrity of intestinal cells and improve the barrier function of the intestinal lining.

Recommended dosage:
The recommended dose ranges from 7 to 14 grams per day.

Posology:
You should take it 2 to 3 times daily, preferably on an empty stomach, in the morning, after exercise, and before bed.

Average action time:
Although the time of onset of action may vary, it usually shows effects after a few weeks to months of continuous use.

Maximum recommended time of continuous use:
There is no established maximum time for continuous use. If it is planned to be used for more than six months in a row, especially in high doses, it is recommended to follow the manufacturer's instructions or consult a specialist.

Licorice

Licorice root has traditionally been used to treat various health problems, including gastritis.

Benefits:
‣ Licorice helps relieve gastritis symptoms due to its anti-inflammatory properties that soothe the stomach lining.

‣ It helps reduce stomach acid production, which can be beneficial.

‣ Some studies have shown that licorice has antioxidant properties that protect stomach cells and help treat gastritis.

Recommended dosage:
The recommended dosage may vary depending on the form of presentation and the concentration of the active ingredient (glycyrrhizinic acid), but generally ranges from 200 to 600 mg

per day.

Posology:
It is recommended to take it, preferably in the morning or during the day, with or without food. It is essential not to consume it on an empty stomach, as it may irritate the stomach. The daily dose can be divided into several intakes to facilitate its absorption.

Average action time:
Although the time of onset of action may vary, it usually affects the digestive system and respiratory health within a few hours of ingestion. Other health problems may require a few weeks to months of continuous use.

Maximum recommended time of continuous use:
A specialist should supervise continued use since prolonged or excessive consumption may cause unwanted side effects, such as electrolyte imbalances or elevated blood pressure. It is recommended to stay within the recommended dose and to consult a physician if use is planned for more than 6 months.

Probiotics

Probiotics are beneficial live microorganisms naturally found in our digestive system. They can be consumed through food or supplements. Their potential to promote gastrointestinal health and balance of the intestinal microbiota has been investigated.

Benefits:
‣ Restoring the balance of the gut microbiota: Gastritis can alter the composition of the gut microbiota, contributing to inflammation and digestive symptoms. Probiotics help restore the balance of beneficial bacteria in the gut, which is valuable for stomach health.

‣ Strengthening the immune system: Probiotics stimulate and strengthen the immune system, reducing inflammation and improving the immune response to gastritis.

‣ Relief of digestive symptoms: Some studies conclude that probiotics help relieve digestive symptoms, such as heartburn, fullness, and alterations in intestinal transit, which may be present in gastritis.

Recommended dosage:
The recommended dosage may vary depending on the type of probiotic strain and individual needs. It is usually between 1 and 10 billion CFU (colony-forming units) per day. Follow the manufacturer's instructions.

Posology:
It is recommended to be taken in the morning or at night. Follow the manufacturer's directions.

Average action time:
Although the onset of action may vary, it usually shows beneficial effects on digestive health and gut microbiota balance after a few weeks of continuous use.

Maximum recommended time of continuous use:
There is no established maximum time for continuous use, as they are safe for consumption for more than six months. It is recommended to follow the manufacturer's directions or consult a specialist if side effects occur or if you wish to use them for more than six months to maintain intestinal health.

Vitamin B12

Vitamin B12 is beneficial for gastritis for several reasons.

Benefits:
‣ Vitamin B12 helps promote the health of the stomach lining by contributing to the regeneration of stomach cells, which is beneficial for those suffering from gastritis.

‣ Vitamin B12 helps reduce symptoms of gastritis by promoting red blood cell production and improving nervous system function, which is beneficial to overall stomach health.

‣ Vitamin B12 deficiency has been associated with an

increased risk of inflammation and damage to the stomach lining, so maintaining adequate levels of vitamin B12 is vital to prevent or treat gastritis.

Recommended dosage:
The recommended dosage may vary depending on individual needs, but generally between 250 to 1000 mcg daily.

Posology:
It should be taken preferably in the morning or during the day. Vitamin B12 is better absorbed when taken with food.

Average action time:
The time of onset of action may vary, but usually shows effect after a few weeks of continuous use.

Maximum recommended time of continuous use:
Continued use is safe in adequate doses. However, please consult your doctor before taking it for over six months.

Zinc

Zinc offers several benefits for gastritis due to its role in gastrointestinal health. It is an essential mineral that plays a vital role in the function and healing of the stomach lining.

Benefits:
▸ Tissue healing and repair: This process is necessary for protein synthesis and the formation of new tissue. It is crucial for healing and restoring the damaged stomach lining.

▸ Strengthening the immune system: It plays a crucial role in the proper function of the immune system. Strengthening the immune system helps protect the stomach lining against infection and reduces inflammation associated with gastritis.

▸ Reduction of inflammation: Zinc has anti-inflammatory properties that help relieve inflammation in the stomach. This is especially beneficial in cases of chronic gastritis, where persistent inflammation can cause discomfort and long-term damage.

Recommended dosage:
The recommended dosage may vary depending on individual needs, but generally between 20 to 35 mg daily.

Posology:
It should be taken preferably during the day, with or without food. It is recommended not to be taken simultaneously with other supplements, such as calcium and iron, as they may interfere with absorption.

Average action time:
The time of onset of action may vary, but usually shows effect after a few weeks of continuous use.

Maximum recommended time of continuous use:
At adequate doses, continued use is safe. However, it is recommended that you consult your doctor if you want to use it for more than 6 months, especially if you have other health problems or if side effects occur. Caution should be exercised with high doses of zinc, as they may cause toxicity.

Strategic Supplement Combinations

When managing gastritis, it is essential to recognize that each supplement provides unique benefits, specifically tailored to alleviate symptoms and enhance gastrointestinal health. Effectively leveraging this variety can play a pivotal role in supporting your recovery.

To adopt a more structured and efficient approach, I recommend implementing a rotational plan for supplement use. Below, you will find carefully curated combinations featuring suggested intake schedules and recommended durations, designed to optimize their benefits and align with your individual needs.

▸ **Phase 1: Combination 1**
Curcumin (morning) and glutamine (afternoon).
Minimum time of use: 4 weeks
Maximum time of use: 8 weeks

> **Phase 2: Combination 2**
Ginger (morning) and chamomile (afternoon).
Minimum time of use: 2 weeks
Maximum time of use: 6 weeks

> **Phase 3: Combination 3**
Probiotics (morning) and licorice (afternoon).
Minimum time of use: 4 weeks
Maximum time of use: 12 weeks

> **Phase 4: Combination 4**
Vitamin B12 (morning) and zinc (afternoon).
Minimum time of use: 6 weeks
Maximum time of use: 10 weeks

This sequence is structured to provide key benefits in the initial combinations, prioritizing the reduction of inflammation and relief of gastritis symptoms. It then transitions to supporting overall gastrointestinal health through the inclusion of probiotics and essential nutrients like vitamin B12 and zinc.

It is important to note that the effectiveness of these supplements may vary from one individual to another.

Adverse Effects, Contraindications, and Interactions

Below is essential information about the potential risks associated with the recommended supplements for gastritis. It is vital to review this section thoroughly before starting their use, as your health should always be the top priority.

Chamomile

> **Side effects**: May cause allergic reactions in some people, especially those sensitive to plants of the Asteraceae family (marigold, chicory, artichoke).

> **Contraindications**: Avoid use if you are pregnant, breast-feeding, allergic to plants of the Asteraceae family, or if you are going to undergo surgery.

> **Interactions**: They may interact with anticoagulant drugs,

sedatives, and diabetes drugs.

Curcumin

▸ **Side effects**: High doses may cause stomach upset, nausea, or diarrhea in some people.

▸ **Contraindications**: Avoid in case of gallstones or people with biliary obstruction.

▸ **Interactions**: May interact with anticoagulant drugs, antiplatelet drugs and drugs for diabetes.

Ginger

▸ **Side effects**: High doses may cause some people heart-burn, diarrhea, or gastrointestinal irritation.

▸ **Contraindications**: These should be avoided in people who have gallstones.

▸ **Interactions**: They may interact with anticoagulants, antiplatelet, and blood pressure drugs.

Glutamine

▸ **Side effects**: Some people may experience stomach upset, bloating, headache, or, in some cases, muscle or joint problems.

▸ **Contraindications**: Avoid in case of severe kidney disease, liver disorders and convulsive disorders.

▸ **Interactions**: Some drugs, such as gamma-aminobutyric acid (GABA) absorption inhibitors, may interact with medications used in chemotherapy. Consult your doctor.

Licorice

▸ **Side effects**: In some people, it may cause high blood pressure, fluid retention, electrolyte imbalances, or hormonal effects.

▸ **Contraindications**: Should be avoided in case of hypertension, heart problems, diabetes, kidney or liver disease, or if you are pregnant.

▸ **Interactions**: Diuretic, corticosteroids, anticoagulants, and blood pressure drugs may interact. Consult your doctor.

Probiotics

▸ **Side effects**: Some people may initially experience mild gastrointestinal discomfort, such as bloating, gas, or stomach upset.

▸ **Contraindications**: It should be avoided in people with a weakened immune system or severe health problems.

▸ **Interactions**: May interact with some immunosuppressive drugs. Consult your doctor.

Vitamin B12

▸ **Side effects**: In very high doses, side effects such as nervousness, anxiety, headache, nausea, or reddening of the skin have been reported.

▸ **Contraindications**: Not suitable for people with severe kidney or liver disease or certain types of cancer.

▸ **Interactions**: It may interact with some drugs, such as proton pump inhibitors, aminoglycoside antibiotics, oral contraceptives, metformin, and folic acid. Consult your doctor.

Zinc

▸ **Side effects**: In some people, it may produce stomach upset, nausea, vomiting, or diarrhea.

▸ **Contraindications**: Not suitable for people with severe kidney or liver disease.

▸ **Interactions**: It may interact with antibiotics, diuretics, oral contraceptives, and osteoporosis drugs. High doses may interfere with the absorption of iron and calcium.

FOODS THAT TRANSFORM

Throughout history, our diet has undergone profoundly radical changes, sharply diverging from the habits of our ancestors. Millions of years ago, early humans shaped their diet around what they could gather or hunt, relying on fresh and raw foods provided by their environment. The emergence of agriculture and livestock farming marked the beginning of a new era of human nutrition, further accelerated by the Industrial Revolution. However, it is important to recognize that while our dietary habits have evolved drastically, our genetics have remained virtually unchanged.

Over time, foods such as dairy products, grains, refined sugars, and vegetable oils were introduced, alongside the rise of intensive meat production. These innovations have made meals more accessible and convenient, yet they have also led to significant changes in nutritional composition. Furthermore, advances in food preservation and culinary techniques gave rise to new methods of storage and preparation, which inevitably impacted food quality.

In recent years, an alarming trend has surfaced: modern diets have become dominated by ultra-processed foods, contributing to the widespread increase in chronic illnesses. Conditions such as obesity, type 2 diabetes, hypertension, and a variety of cardiovascular and digestive disorders have all been closely linked to this dietary shift. Why is this happening? Primarily because ultra-processed foods are heavily laden with refined carbohydrates, unhealthy fats, added sugars, chemical additives, and low-quality vegetable oils. Even meats and other animal products from intensive farming systems are often filled with substances harmful to health. These processed foods have largely replaced traditional diets, which were built on fresh and natural ingredients, disrupting the equilibrium that once fostered optimal well-being among our ancestors.

Nonetheless, there is hope for reversing this trend: small yet thoughtful changes to our eating habits can have a significant impact on our health. Returning to a balanced, nutrient-rich way of eating, centered on fresh, whole foods, is essential for establishing a strong foundation for wellness. Integrating fruits, vegetables, root vegetables, legumes, nuts, and seeds into the diet is a powerful step toward revitalizing the way we nourish ourselves. Despite this, one major challenge persists: the consumption of these natural, unprocessed foods remains astonishingly low in many parts of the world.

Choosing a lifestyle rooted in mindful eating not only helps prevent diseases associated with poor dietary habits but also rejuvenates the body and mind. By prioritizing real, wholesome foods and cutting back on ultra-processed options, we can cultivate a healthier, more balanced, and fulfilling life. Now is the time to rediscover the transformative power of a healthy diet–not as a form of restriction, but as an act of self-care. Your health deserves that commitment!

Understanding the Link Between Nutrition and Health

How often have you asked yourself if what you eat truly supports your well-being? The relationship between nutrition and health is far deeper than we commonly realize. Understanding which foods promote wellness and which ones to avoid, tailored to your specific needs, is a powerful step toward improving your quality of life. This isn't a new concept; it has been examined and revered for centuries. Since ancient times, cultures around the world have recognized the therapeutic value of nutrition as a means to heal, strengthen, and sustain the body, leaving us a profound legacy of wisdom.

Traditional medical systems–such as Traditional Chinese Medicine, the practices of ancient Egypt, Greece, and Rome, Ayurveda in India, and indigenous healing methods across the Americas–delved into the restorative potential of natural foods. These practices emphasized the idea that food does much more than nourish; it can protect, alleviate discomfort, and even heal the body.

For many years, these age-old principles were often dismissed by conventional medicine as unscientific. Yet, modern research has gradually confirmed what our ancestors intuitively understood: the foods we eat directly affect not only our physical health but also our emotional well-being. Today, scientific studies continue to uncover compounds in food with therapeutic properties that help prevent diseases, reduce symptoms, and promote overall health.

Researchers have spent decades analyzing how certain foods strengthen the body and protect against chronic illnesses, identifying dietary patterns in populations with low disease rates that differ significantly from those in less healthy communities. These studies reveal the decisive role specific nutrients play in promoting vitality and longevity, with certain foods offering unique benefits such as anti-inflammatory properties to manage joint pain and chronic discomfort, antimicrobial effects to bolster immune defenses, anticoagulant actions to support cardiovascular health, antihypertensive abilities to regulate blood pressure, and mood-enhancing compounds that alleviate anxiety while fostering emotional resilience.

What you choose to eat influences not only your daily energy but also your capacity to recover, fend off illness, and pursue a fulfilling life. On the flip side, a poor diet or reliance on unhealthy foods can exacerbate health problems, intensify symptoms, and undermine overall well-being.

The encouraging part? Every day offers the chance to make dietary choices that lead to better health. While external factors like pollution or environmental changes may remain out of your control, your diet is a fundamental tool for self-care. Each ingredient on your plate carries the potential to positively impact both your physical and mental health.

Learning which foods are best for your unique needs–and understanding which ones may harm your health–can empower you to find balance and achieve a healthier, more vibrant lifestyle. Nutrition, humanity's earliest form of medicine, is not just a pathway to wellness but also a connection to our roots, equipping us for a future filled with possibilities.

I invite you to explore how nutrition can become your strongest ally in easing ailments, building resilience, and fostering happiness. Are you ready to embrace this journey of discovery and transformation? Your well-being is within your control, and every meal is a chance to create a life of greater health and vitality. Start today: Nourish your body, refresh your mind, and live fully.

Cooking Techniques

Healthy cooking is essential for everyone, especially after the age of 40. Below are various cooking techniques along with their related health benefits and potential risks.

Healthier Ways of Cooking

▸ **Steaming**: Steaming is an excellent method for preserving nutrients, as it does not require the use of additional fats. It helps keep food tender and juicy while being a gentle cooking technique that does not contribute to the formation of harmful compounds.

▸ **Oven roasting**: Oven roasting is a healthy option that does not require added oils. Foods like vegetables, fish, and chicken can be roasted in the oven to create nutritious and flavorful meals.

▸ **Light sautéing**: This method involves quickly cooking food over high heat with a small amount of healthy oil, such as olive or coconut oil. Light sautéing helps maintain the food's texture and nutrients while cooking it efficiently.

▸ **Boiling**: Boiling is a healthy cooking method, particularly for vegetables. It preserves nutrients and creates a tender texture. However, it is crucial to avoid overcooking to minimize nutrient loss.

▸ **Baking**: Baking is an excellent way to prepare food without the need for added oils. Foods like fish, poultry, vegetables, and whole grains can be baked for healthy and flavorful dishes.

Less Healthy Ways of Cooking

▸ **Frying**: Frying involves submerging food in hot oil, which significantly increases its saturated fat and calorie content. Additionally, frying at high temperatures can produce harmful compounds that pose health risks.

▸ **Breading and battering**: Coating food in breading or batter increases its calorie and fat content. These coatings can absorb more oil during cooking, resulting in a less nutritious meal.

▸ **Creamy sauces and dressings**: Cream-based sauces and dressings often contain high levels of saturated fat and excess calories. These can contribute to inflammation and exacerbate pain.

▸ **Grilling at high temperatures**: Cooking food on the grill at high heat can generate harmful compounds, such as polycyclic aromatic hydrocarbons (PAHs) and heterocyclic amines (HCAs), which have been associated with an increased cancer risk. Additionally, grilled meats can produce inflammatory substances.

Remember, the way you cook food significantly impacts its nutritional value and its overall effects on your health. Choosing healthy cooking methods ensures you maximize the benefits of your meals while reducing potential negative effects.

Tips to Prevent and Ease Gastritis

Gastritis can be challenging for your digestive system, but adopting a few simple and positive habits can make a big difference. Whether you're looking to prevent it or manage symptoms, these recommendations can help you achieve a healthier stomach and improve your overall well-being:

▸ **Enjoy 4 to 5 light meals a day**. Keep meals small and manageable to support healthy digestion and minimize acidity or gas.

‣ **Stick to regular mealtimes**. Consistency allows your stomach to better regulate digestive processes.

‣ **Finish dinner 2 to 3 hours before bedtime**. This gives your body enough time to digest food before you lie down.

‣ **Stay hydrated with at least 1.5 liters of water daily**. Drink water between meals rather than during them. If you must, sip small amounts, like half a glass, while eating.

‣ **Eat slowly and chew your food thoroughly**. Rushing through meals or not chewing enough places extra strain on your stomach.

‣ **Stick to foods at moderate temperatures**. Avoid extremes —foods and drinks that are too hot or too cold can irritate your stomach lining.

‣ **Cut back on fried and high-fat foods**. These are harder to digest and may aggravate symptoms.

‣ **Add fiber to your diet**. Eat whole grains, vegetables, legumes, and fruits to promote a healthy digestive system.

‣ **Handle raw foods with care**. Reduce your intake of raw meat or fish, like carpaccio or sushi, to lower your risk of infections like Helicobacter pylori.

‣ **Always check food quality**. Avoid eating anything spoiled or past its expiration date to protect your stomach.

‣ **Cook food using gentle methods**. Choose boiling, baking, steaming, grilling, or broiling over frying.

‣ **Avoid irritants like coffee, tea, soda, alcohol, and spicy foods**. These can inflame the stomach and worsen symptoms.

‣ **Reduce high-fat foods**. Limit red meat, full-fat dairy, and fried items. Instead, choose lean meats like skinless poultry or turkey and low-fat fish such as salmon or trout.

‣ **Choose low-fat dairy.** Options like skim milk or low-fat yogurt are easier on your stomach.

‣ **Watch your salt intake.** Excess salt can increase stomach acidity. Enhance flavors with gentle herbs and mild spices instead.

‣ **Incorporate antioxidant-rich foods.** Fruits and vegetables can help reduce inflammation and support your stomach lining.

‣ **Eat more soluble fiber.** Foods like oats, apples, and legumes help regulate digestion and reduce acidity.

‣ **Avoid fast food and oversized meals.** Opt for smaller portions, chew your food thoroughly, and eat mindfully for easier digestion.

‣ **Elevate your bed if you experience reflux.** Raising the head of your bed at night prevents stomach acid from reaching your esophagus.

By embracing these habits, you can support your stomach health and lead a more comfortable, symptom-free life. Take it one step at a time–your body will thank you!

Healing Foods, according to TCM

According to the principles of ancient Traditional Chinese Medicine, certain foods possess therapeutic properties that can help alleviate or improve the symptoms of gastritis. Below is a detailed list of the most noteworthy ones:

‣ **Apple cider vinegar:**

Apple cider vinegar contains malic acid, which benefits digestion and balances the stomach's pH. Two teaspoons of it should be mixed in a glass of water and consumed twice or thrice daily.

▸ **Grape** (Vitis vinifera):
Eating raw black grapes is beneficial for gastritis. You should consume half to one kilogram daily for one to three days without eating other food. The grapes can also be consumed as juice, which contains alkalizing and detoxifying organic elements.

▸ **Spinach** (Spinacia oleracea):
Spinach detoxifies the intestinal tract, restores pH, and calms inflammation. It can be consumed raw in salads or as juice. Mix 6 parts spinach with 10 parts carrot juice and drink half a liter to a liter daily.

▸ **Yogurt:**
It is essential to consume only natural yogurt without sugar to treat gastritis.

FOR CHRONIC GASTRITIS

▸ **Apple** (Malus pumila):
Ingredients: 1 apple. Eat it after meals, well washed.
Precautions: According to TCM, excessive apple consumption may cause abdominal bloating due to its fresh nature.

▸ **Grape** (Vitis vinifera):
Ingredients: red wine. Take 15 ml of red wine 2 or 3 times a day.

▸ **Mandarin** (Citrus reticulata):
Preparation: Scour 30 grams of dried tangerine peel on a griddle. Then grind it and mix 6 grams of the powdered peel with water and brown sugar. Take twice a day, 15-30 minutes before eating, on an empty stomach.
Precautions: According to TCM, although mandarin is fresh, excessive consumption can quickly increase internal fire. Therefore, it should not be consumed in abundance if you have mouth sores, dry and hard defecation, cough caused by cold factors, or phlegm.

▸ **Quail** (Coturnix coturnix):
Preparation: Cook 1 to 3 quail eggs in boiling milk. Consume in the morning.

▸ **Sugar cane** (Saccharum officinarum):

Preparation 1: Mix 100 ml of sugar cane juice with 100 ml of grape wine. Take in the morning and evening.

Preparation 2: Mix 150 ml of sugar cane juice with 5 grams of ginger juice. Take on an empty stomach in the morning.

Precautions: According to Traditional Chinese Medicine (TCM), sugarcane should not be consumed if it has a yellowish color, sour taste, fermented odor, or is rotten, as it may cause intoxication. In addition, people suffering from weakness or cold in the spleen or stomach should be cautious when consuming it raw due to its cold nature.

FOR GASTRODUODENAL ULCER

▸ **Mandarin** (Citrus reticulata):

Ingredients: 100 grams of dried tangerine peel, 100 grams of licorice, and 100 grams of honey.

Preparation: Soak the licorice and tangerine peel in water for a few hours. Then, cook them for 20 minutes and extract the juice. Repeat this process three times. Mix the juice and simmer it until it becomes a thick syrup. Add double the amount of honey and turn off the heat when it starts to boil. Take 30 grams, mixed with warm water, two times a day.

FOR CHRONIC GASTRITIS, ANTRAL GASTRITIS AND GASTRODUODENAL ULCER

▸ **Rice** (Oryza sativa):

Ingredients: glutinous rice.

Preparation: Prepare a very well-cooked rice soup. Take it daily.

Ingredients: 100 grams of non-glutinous round rice and ginger juice. *Preparation*: Toast the rice in a frying pan until it burns. Grind the rice into a fine powder. Take 5 grams of the powder mixed with ginger juice before meals.

FOR GASTRITIS ACCOMPANIED BY VOMITING

▸ **Garlic** (Allium sativum):

Ingredients: 2 heads of garlic and honey. To prepare, cook the garlic and mix it with the honey and boiled water.

Precautions: According to TCM, garlic should not be consumed in excess for a long time (more than three months), as it can increase internal heat and affect eyesight. Abusing garlic is also not recommended in cases of stomach dysfunction.

Natural Remedies for H. Pylori

Presented below are some of the most effective natural treatments for combating this bacteria. Follow the recommended duration for each treatment, and afterward, consult a doctor to verify that the infection has been completely eliminated.

Broccoli

Ingredients: 1 broccoli, a pinch of sea salt, and 250 ml of boiled water. *Preparation*: Wash the broccoli well. Process it in a blender with the boiled water and the pinch of salt, leaving a homogeneous mixture without lumps. Please take it in the morning on an empty stomach and at night before sleeping for 1 or 2 months.

Note: broccoli taken in this form has no adverse effects or interactions.

Ginger

This root has bactericidal properties that will help you eradicate it. You can take it for a maximum of two months.

Infusion: 1 or 2 grams of peeled ginger and 1 cup of water. Boil the water with the ginger for 5-10 minutes. Strain and drink 1 or 2 times daily, at least 1 hour before eating.

Ginger can also be eaten raw or added to food.

Note: This book's "Medicinal Plants" chapter discusses this plant's adverse effects and interactions. Please read it before taking it.

Lemon Verbena Essential Oil

Add 15 to 20 drops of the essential oil diluted in half a glass of water after each meal for 1 week.

You can also prepare an infusion from the leaves of the lemon verbena plant. In this case, use three or four leaves. Boil water, remove it from the heat, and add the leaves. Cover and let it steep for five minutes. Take it after meals for two weeks.

Licorice

To solve this problem, consume it for a maximum of 2 months. You have several ways to take it:

Decoction: 1 teaspoon of dried root and 1 glass of water. Heat the water. When it starts to boil, add the licorice and let it cook for 10-15 minutes. Remove from heat and let it stand for 10-15 minutes more. Sweeten with stevia. Drink 2 or 3 cups a day.

Cold licorice infusion: Ingredients: 1-2 teaspoons of licorice root. Preparation: Soak licorice in a bowl of cold water for 12 hours. Drink a cup every day for 4 to 8 weeks.

Infusion: 1 small spoonful of crushed dried root and 1 glass of water. Boil the water and remove it from the heat. Add the licorice and cover for 10 minutes. Drink 2 or 3 cups a day.

You can also suck or bite the root directly.

Lemon and Gastritis: Myth or Remedy?

The relationship between lemons and gastritis has been a hot topic of debate in health and nutrition circles. To unravel this controversy, it's crucial to examine the following key aspects:

▸ **Properties of lemon**

Lemon is a citrus fruit widely known for its high vitamin C and antioxidant content. Its acidic pH is generally around 2 to 3, which makes it quite acidic compared to other foods. This level of acidity has generated controversy regarding its impact on gastric conditions such as gastritis.

In addition to vitamin C, lemons contain bioactive compounds such as flavonoids, which have anti-inflammatory and antioxidant properties. In folk medicine, lemons have been used to detoxify the body, improve digestion, and strengthen the immune system.

▸ **Controversy: Does lemon aggravate or relieve gastritis?**

The controversy is whether lemon consumption can aggravate or alleviate gastritis symptoms. Some health professionals argue that lemon's acidity may further irritate the inflamed gastric mucosa, worsening gastritis symptoms. This perspective is based on the notion that acidic foods may increase gastric acid production, exacerbating inflammation and pain.

On the other hand, some argue that, despite its external acidity, lemon has an alkalizing effect on the body once metabolized. According to this theory, lemon consumption could potentially balance the body's pH and thus help soothe the gastric mucosa. In addition, the antioxidants and flavonoids present in lemon could have a protective and regenerative effect on the stomach lining.

▸ Scientific evidence
Scientific evidence on the impact of lemon on gastritis is limited and often contradictory. Some studies have explored the effects of citrus fruits in general on gastric health, but few have explicitly focused on lemon. The lack of high-quality, controlled studies makes it difficult to draw definitive conclusions.

A study published in a medical journal investigated the effect of different acidic foods on people with gastritis and found that some people experienced increased symptoms after consuming citrus fruits, including lemon. However, these effects were not universal and varied significantly among individuals.

On the other hand, research on the anti-inflammatory effects of flavonoids concludes that there may be potential benefits in consuming foods rich in these compounds for inflammatory conditions, although direct application to gastritis requires further investigation.

▸ Individual considerations
People with gastritis can respond widely to lemon consumption. Factors such as the underlying cause of gastritis, other health conditions, and individual sensitivity to acidic foods are crucial in determining how a person may react to lemon.

▸ Alternatives to lemon
For those who find that lemon worsens their gastritis symptoms, some alternatives can offer similar benefits without heartburn. Foods such as papaya, which contains natural digestive enzymes, or ginger, known for its anti-inflammatory properties, can improve digestion and reduce gastric inflammation.

▸ Conclusion
The debate surrounding lemons and gastritis highlights the

intricate relationship between diet and digestive health. While lemons may provide benefits for some, they can worsen symptoms in others.

Given these individual differences, it's essential to pay attention to your body's response and tailor your diet to suit your specific needs when managing gastritis.

Beneficial Foods and Beverages

Following a proper diet is crucial for relieving gastritis symptoms and supporting the healing of the gastric lining. Here is a selection of foods and beverages recommended for their beneficial properties:

- **Fiber-rich foods**: High-fiber foods can help relieve gastritis symptoms and promote digestive health. Fresh fruits and vegetables, such as apples, pears, bananas, carrots and spinach, are excellent sources of fiber. In addition, whole grains, such as brown rice, oatmeal and whole wheat bread, are also healthy choices.

- **Lean proteins**: Choose lean protein sources such as chicken, turkey, fish and tofu. These proteins are more accessible to digest than fatty meats and can help repair and regenerate the stomach lining.

- **Low-fat dairy**: Low-fat dairy products, such as low-fat yogurt and cottage cheese, may be well tolerated for gastritis. These foods provide protein and calcium, but check for flavors or additives that may irritate the stomach.

- **Foods rich in omega-3**: Omega-3 fatty acids are anti-inflammatory and may benefit gastritis. Oily fish, such as salmon, tuna, and sardines, are excellent sources of omega-3. You can also incorporate chia seeds, walnuts and olive oil into your diet.

- **Soft and easy-to-digest foods**: During episodes of gastritis, it is advisable to eat soft and easy-to-digest foods. Smooth soups, vegetable purees, fruit compotes and porridges can provide nutrients without burdening the stomach.

▸ **Herbal infusions**: Some herbal infusions, taken after eating, help relieve gastritis symptoms. Chamomile, ginger, and licorice tea are soothing and help reduce inflammation and stomach discomfort.

▸ **Water**: Staying well hydrated is essential for good digestive health. Water can dilute stomach acid and help relieve symptoms of gastritis. Drink water at room temperature and avoid hot or cold drinks, which can trigger discomfort.

▸ **Probiotics**: Probiotic-rich foods, such as probiotic yogurt, kefir and sauerkraut, contain beneficial bacteria that can promote a healthy balance in the digestive system. Probiotics help reduce inflammation and improve the health of the stomach mucosa.

To simplify this process, consider maintaining a food journal. Document your daily consumption and assess how it impacts your digestion and overall well-being. This habit can empower you to make more informed choices on your path to optimal digestive health.

Harmful Foods and Beverages

To simplify this process, consider maintaining a food journal. Document your daily consumption and assess how it impacts your digestion and overall well-being. This habit can empower you to make more informed choices on your path to optimal digestive health.

▸ **Fatty foods**: High-fat foods, such as fried foods, fatty meats and full-fat dairy products, can increase stomach acid production and worsen gastritis symptoms. Instead of fried, it is advisable to opt for leaner options, such as lean meats, low-fat dairy products, and baked or steamed preparations.

▸ **Acidic foods**: Acidic foods, such as citrus fruits (lemons, oranges, grapefruit), tomatoes, and their derivatives (tomato sauces, juices), can irritate the stomach lining and increase acidity. Therefore, they are suggested to be limited in consumption and replaced with less acidic alternatives.

▸ **Caffeinated beverages**: Coffee, tea, soft drinks and energy drinks containing caffeine can increase stomach acidity and worsen gastritis symptoms. It is advisable to limit or avoid their consumption and opt for caffeine-free alternatives, such as herbal teas or water.

▸ **Alcoholic beverages**: Alcohol can irritate the stomach lining and increase stomach acid production, which can exacerbate the symptoms of gastritis. It is recommended that alcohol be avoided entirely during the treatment of gastritis.

▸ **Spicy foods**: Very spicy foods, such as chili, curry, and hot sauces, can irritate the stomach and cause symptoms of heartburn and discomfort. It is best to avoid highly spicy foods and opt for milder, less irritating options.

▸ **Processed foods**: Processed foods, such as fast foods, sausages and convenience foods, often contain high levels of saturated fats, additives and preservatives, which can trigger or worsen stomach inflammation. It is suggested that fresh and natural foods be prioritized over processed options.

▸ **Citrus foods**: In addition to the citrus fruits mentioned above, it is essential to avoid other acidic foods, such as vinegar, pineapple and berries. These foods can irritate the stomach lining and increase gastric acid production.

▸ **Foods rich in spices**: Strong spices, such as capsicum, black pepper, garlic and onion, can trigger heartburn symptoms and discomfort in people with gastritis. It is recommended that they be reduced or avoided altogether.

▸ **Fried and fatty foods**: Fried foods, such as French fries, empanadas and battered foods, can be challenging to digest and aggravate stomach inflammation. In addition, fatty foods, such as fatty meats and full-fat dairy products, can increase stomach acid production and worsen gastritis symptoms.

▸ **Carbonated beverages**: Carbonated beverages, such as soda and sparkling water, can cause bloating and increase stomach pressure, aggravating gastritis symptoms. It is better to opt for still water or other non-carbonated beverages.

▸ **Chocolate and cocoa products**: Chocolate contains caffeine and fats, which can trigger heartburn symptoms and worsen gastritis in some people. In addition, dark chocolate and cocoa powder are rich in stimulant compounds, such as theobromine, which can increase stomach acid production.

▸ **Foods high in salt**: Salty foods, such as processed foods, fast foods and snacks, can irritate the stomach lining and aggravate gastritis symptoms. Reducing salt intake and avoiding fresh foods with no added salt is recommended.

It is crucial to remember that each individual may respond differently to certain foods and beverages. What worsens symptoms for one person may cause no discomfort for another.

Gastritis Support: Easy and Tasty Recipes

Do you struggle with gastritis and need delicious options that won't upset your stomach? Here, you'll find quick, easy, and nutritious recipes designed to nurture your stomach without giving up the pleasure of eating. However, remember that every body is unique–pay attention to your own needs and adjust these recipes to suit your preferences and tolerances. Your well-being is always the top priority!

Breakfast Options

1. Oatmeal bowl: Prepare oatmeal with water or low-fat milk. Add sliced banana, fresh berries, and a tablespoon of honey.

2. Avocado toast: Toast a slice of whole wheat bread and spread it with mashed avocado. Add a little salt and pepper to taste.

3. Yogurt with fruit: Choose a low-fat yogurt with no added sugar. Add pieces of soft fruit, such as bananas or mango.

4. Whole-grain toast with sugar-free jam: Toast a slice of whole-grain bread and spread it with a sugar-free jam, such as berries.

5. Banana and ginger smoothie: Blend a ripe banana, half a glass of unsweetened almond milk, a pinch of grated fresh ginger, and a tablespoon of chia seeds.

6. Scrambled eggs with spinach: Cook two egg whites in a nonstick skillet and add a handful of fresh spinach–season with salt and pepper to taste.

7. Oatmeal pancakes: Mix ground oats, egg whites, low-fat milk, and a pinch of cinnamon. Cook pancakes in a non-stick pan and serve with fresh fruit.

8. Pineapple-Coconut Smoothie: Blend fresh pineapple, unsweetened coconut milk, low-fat Greek yogurt and ice. Add a little honey for more sweetness.

9. Rye toast with salmon: Toast a slice of rye bread and spread it with low-fat cream cheese. Add slices of smoked salmon and some fresh dill.

Remember that it is advisable to eat small portions and eat slowly to facilitate digestion.

Lunch Creations

1. Baked chicken with steamed vegetables: Bake chicken breasts seasoned with mild herbs and serve with steamed vegetables, such as broccoli, carrots and zucchini.

2. Brown rice with grilled fish: Prepare brown rice and serve it with grilled fish fillets seasoned with lemon* and mild spices.

3. Quinoa and vegetable salad: Mix cooked quinoa with cucumber, tomato, bell pepper, and spinach leaves. Dress with light olive oil and lemon dressing*.

4. Vegetable soup: Prepare a mild, comforting soup with low-fat chicken broth, carrots, celery, squash and a little white rice.

5. Baked turkey with mashed potatoes: Bake a breast seasoned with mild herbs and serve it with light, smooth mashed potatoes.

6. Egg white omelet with spinach: Make an omelet with egg whites and add sautéed spinach. Serve with a slice of whole wheat bread.

7. Banana and oatmeal smoothie: Blend ripe banana, oatmeal, plain nonfat yogurt and a little honey in a blender for a smooth and nutritious smoothie.

8. Pumpkin and carrot puree: Cook the pumpkin and carrots, then mash them to a smooth puree. Add a little ginger for extra flavor.

9. Baked fish with lemon slices* and herbs: Bake fish fillets with lemon slices* and mild herbs such as parsley. Serve with a portion of white rice.

10. Chicken and avocado salad: Mix grilled chicken pieces with avocado, spinach leaves, and cherry tomatoes, then dress with a light olive oil and lemon dressing.

11. Baked salmon with asparagus: Bake salmon fillets with lemon* and mild herbs, such as dill, and serve with steamed or baked asparagus.

12. Turkey and avocado tacos: Fill corn tortillas or lettuce wraps with ground turkey cooked with mild spices. Add sliced avocado and a little mild salsa.

13. Banana and strawberry smoothie: Blend ripe banana, strawberries, plain nonfat yogurt and a little honey in a blender for a smooth and refreshing smoothie.

14. Mashed potatoes and carrots: Cook and mash potatoes and carrots to make a smooth, comforting mash. Add a little vegetable broth for extra flavor.

15. Scrambled eggs with spinach: Prepare scrambled eggs

with fresh spinach and a little soft cheese. Serve with a slice of toasted whole wheat bread.

16. Rice with chicken and vegetables: Cook brown rice with grilled chicken pieces and vegetables such as broccoli, carrots and peas–season with mild herbs.

17. Apple and pear puree: Cook apples and pears until soft, then mash them to make a smooth, natural puree. If desired, add a touch of cinnamon.

18. Grilled chicken breast with quinoa: Season grilled chicken breast with mild herbs and serve it with cooked quinoa and steamed broccoli.

19. Tuna and avocado salad: Mix canned tuna, avocado, tomato, cucumber and greens. Dress with a light olive oil dressing and a squeeze of lemon*.

20. Lentils with carrots and zucchini: Prepare a mild stew of cooked lentils, carrots, and zucchini. Add crushed tomatoes and season with mild herbs.

21. Turkey in yogurt and herb sauce: Cook turkey strips with a mild natural yogurt sauce and herbs such as cilantro. Serve with white or brown rice.

22. Banana and spinach smoothie: Blend a ripe banana, fresh spinach, plain nonfat yogurt and a little honey for a nutrient-rich smoothie.

23. Broccoli and cauliflower puree: Cook broccoli and cauliflower until tender, then mash them into a smooth, nutritious puree. Add a little vegetable broth for extra flavor.

24. Spinach and cheese omelet: Prepare an omelet with egg whites, fresh spinach and low-fat cheese. Serve with a soft cucumber and tomato salad.

25. Steamed salmon with dill sauce: Cook steamed salmon fillets with lemon slices and a mild dill-and-lemon sauce. Serve with brown rice.

26. Sweet potato and carrot puree: Cook sweet potatoes and carrots until soft, then mash them to make a creamy, comforting puree. Add a touch of ginger for extra flavor.

27. Turkey breast with zucchini puree: Bake a breast seasoned with mild herbs and serve with a soft and light zucchini puree.

28. Chickpea and tomato salad: Mix chickpeas with tomato, cucumber, bell pepper and onion. Dress with olive oil, a pinch of cumin, and a squeeze of lemon*.

29. Curried vegetable rice: Cook brown rice and mix it with steamed vegetables, such as carrots, peas and zucchini, seasoned with a mild curry sauce.

30. Grilled chicken with cucumber salad: Grill chicken breasts with mild herbs and serve with a fresh salad and a squeeze of lemon*.

31. Banana and almond smoothie: Blend a ripe banana, almonds, plain nonfat yogurt and a little honey in a blender for a creamy and nutritious smoothie.

(*Refer to the chapter "Foods That Transform", section "Lemon and Gastritis: Myth or Remedy?" for more information).

Snacks

1. Banana and spinach smoothie: Blend one ripe banana, one cup of fresh spinach, half a glass of low-fat milk, and one tablespoon of honey.

2. Rice pancakes with almond butter: Spread brown rice pancakes with a thin layer of natural almond butter.

3. Apple slices with cottage cheese: Slice an apple and

combine it with low-fat cottage cheese.

4. Carrot sticks with hummus: Cut carrots into sticks and serve with homemade or store-bought hummus without spice.

5. Turkey and avocado rolls: Wrap a slice of low-fat turkey around a slice of avocado. If desired, add a little light mustard.

6. Fruit gelatin: Prepare sugar-free gelatin according to package directions and add pieces of soft fruit, such as peaches in syrup or strawberries.

7. Handful of nuts: Nuts are a healthy snack option. Choose natural, unsalted nuts and enjoy them in small amounts.

8. Lettuce rolls with chicken: Wrap grilled chicken slices in lettuce leaves, then add cucumber and carrot slices. Season with olive oil and a little lemon*.

9. Applesauce: Cook peeled and diced apples with water and cinnamon until soft. Mash into a smooth compote and enjoy cold or warm.

Dinner Ideas

1. Baked chicken breast with steamed vegetables: Bake a chicken breast seasoned with mild herbs and serve it with steamed vegetables such as broccoli, carrots and zucchini.

2. Grilled salmon with mashed potatoes and spinach: Grill a salmon fillet with a bit of lemon* and serve it with soft mashed potatoes and cooked spinach.

3. Quinoa salad with chicken and avocado: Mix cooked quinoa with grilled chicken pieces, sliced avocado, tomato and cucumber. Dress with olive oil and a squeeze of lemon*.

4. Egg white omelet with spinach and mushrooms: Prepare an omelet with egg whites, fresh spinach and mushrooms. Serve with a soft cucumber and tomato salad.

5. Whole wheat pasta with chicken and steamed vegetables: Cook whole wheat pasta and mix it with grilled chicken strips and steamed vegetables such as peppers, broccoli and carrots. Dress with a bit of olive oil.

6. Vegetable and chicken soup: Prepare a mild vegetable soup with pieces of cooked chicken, such as carrots, zucchini, celery and onion. You can season with mild herbs such as parsley.

7. Baked fish with roasted vegetables: Bake white fish fillets with a bit of lemon* and a pinch of pepper, and accompany them with roasted vegetables such as peppers, eggplant and zucchini.

8. Quinoa salad with smoked salmon: Mix and cook with smoked salmon chunks, avocado, cherry tomatoes, and cucumber. Dress with a light olive oil vinaigrette and a squeeze of lemon*.

9. Chickpea puree with grilled chicken: Mash chickpeas with garlic, lemon juice, and cumin to make a smooth puree. Serve with grilled chicken breasts and a fresh salad.

10. Turkey breast rolls with spinach and cheese: Wrap fresh spinach and low-fat cheese in a turkey breast and bake until cooked. Serve with a green salad.

11. Lentil curry with brown rice: Prepare a mild lentil curry with tomato, turmeric and ginger and serve it with brown rice.

12. Chicken and apple salad: Mix grilled chicken chunks with diced apple, walnuts and lettuce. Dress with a honey mustard vinaigrette.

13. Baked turkey with pumpkin puree: Prepare a baked turkey breast with mild herbs and serve with a smooth pumpkin and carrot puree.

14. Quinoa and avocado salad: Mix cooked quinoa with diced avocado, cherry tomatoes, cucumber and green leaves.

Dress with olive oil and a squeeze of lemon*.

15. Zucchini and carrot soup: Cook zucchini and carrots in vegetable broth, then puree to make a smooth, comforting soup.

16. Chicken in yogurt sauce: Grill chicken breasts and serve them with a mild sauce of natural yogurt, a little lemon juice*, and herbs such as cilantro.

17. Chickpea and cucumber salad: Mix cooked chickpeas with cucumber, tomato, onion, and bell pepper. Dress with olive oil, a squeeze of lemon, and a little cumin.

18. Sweet potato and carrot puree with baked salmon: Prepare a creamy sweet potato and carrot puree and serve it with a baked salmon fillet, dill, and a little lemon*.

19. Zucchini and cheese omelet: Prepare an omelet with grated zucchini, low-fat cheese and fresh herbs. Serve with a soft salad of lettuce and cucumber.

20. Whole wheat pasta with tomato sauce and chicken: Cook whole wheat pasta and mix it with a mild tomato sauce, grilled chicken pieces and fresh spinach.

21. Chicken and vegetable soup: This comforting soup uses chicken broth, cooked chicken pieces, carrots, celery and onion. Brown rice adds more substance.

22. Baked hake fillet with broccoli puree: Bake a hake fillet with a bit of lemon* and herbs, and accompany it with a soft broccoli puree.

23. Lentil salad with roasted vegetables: Mix cooked lentils with roasted vegetables such as peppers, eggplant and zucchini. Dress with olive oil.

24. Corn tortillas with shredded chicken and avocado: Prepare corn tortillas filled with shredded chicken, sliced avocado, and some fresh cilantro.

25. Baked salmon with asparagus and potatoes: Bake salmon fillets with dill and a squeeze of lemon*, and serve with steamed asparagus and baked potato wedges.

26. Quinoa salad with grilled vegetables: Mix cooked quinoa with grilled vegetables such as zucchini, peppers and mushrooms. Dress with a light vinaigrette of fresh herbs and a squeeze of lemon*.

27. Chicken breast stuffed with spinach and feta cheese: Stuff chicken breasts with fresh spinach and feta cheese, bake, and serve with a green salad.

28. Whole wheat pasta with steamed chicken and broccoli: Prepare whole wheat pasta and mix it with grilled chicken pieces and steamed broccoli. Dress with olive oil and garlic.

29. Chickpea salad with tuna and cucumber: Combine cooked chickpeas with canned tuna, diced cucumber, and peppers. Dress with fresh herbs and a squeeze of lemon*.

30. Creamy pumpkin and carrot soup: Cook pumpkin and carrots in vegetable broth, puree to a creamy texture, and add a touch of ginger.

31. Turkey burgers with fresh salad: Prepare burgers with mild herbs and garlic and serve them with a fresh salad of lettuce, tomato and cucumber. To make the dish lighter, substitute lettuce leaves for the bread.

(*Refer to the chapter "Foods That Transform", section "Lemon and Gastritis: Myth or Remedy?" for more information).

Always customize the recipes to suit your individual needs and tolerances, as your well-being is the top priority. I hope these suggestions prove helpful, delicious, and inspire you to enjoy balanced meals that aid in managing your gastritis and acid reflux effectively. Savor every bite, and take care of your health!

JUICES AND SMOOTHIES

Raw foods, often referred to as "living" foods, are an exceptional source of vitamins, minerals, fiber, trace elements, enzymes, and other vital compounds that support overall health. Incorporating these nutrient-rich foods into your daily diet not only aids in disease prevention but also alleviates symptoms of various health conditions, slows down the aging process, balances gut flora, and enhances energy levels and vitality.

While salads, whole fruits, and nuts are excellent raw food options, one of the easiest and most convenient ways to ensure regular intake is by preparing homemade juices, smoothies, and shakes. These beverages serve as a delicious and practical alternative for individuals who may not enjoy consuming fruits and vegetables directly, making it easier to include these essential nutrients in their diet.

In today's world, where ultra-processed foods and toxins have become increasingly prevalent, the need for natural, nutrient-dense foods is more crucial than ever. Raw foods play a vital role in supporting detoxification, maintaining health, and restoring balance to the body.

Many people tend to prepare their juices and smoothies using only fruits, often overlooking the incredible health benefits vegetables and leafy greens provide. Adding these to your recipes not only increases variety but also significantly boosts their nutritional value, enhancing their antioxidant, remineralizing, toning, and alkalizing properties. These qualities help maintain the body's balance, rejuvenate cells, and promote overall well-being. Additionally, vegetables and greens lower the glycemic index, improve satiety, and maximize the health benefits of these preparations.

However, it is crucial to understand that most store-bought juices are far from healthy options. These commercial products are often loaded with excessive added sugars, artificial sweeteners, preservatives, and harmful chemical additives. Furthermore, the pasteurization processes used during production strip away essential vitamins and enzymes, rendering them nutritionally deficient. The high level of refinement also removes fiber, a vital component of whole foods. In many cases, these juices contain only minimal amounts of actual fruit, making them highly processed and lacking true nutritional value.

One major concern with many juices and smoothies is their high glycemic index, which can cause blood sugar spikes, lead to weight gain, and contribute to long-term metabolic imbalances. To truly enjoy healthy and nourishing beverages, the best approach is to prepare them at home using fresh, natural, and high-quality ingredients. Homemade juices and smoothies are packed with nutrients that provide genuine benefits for your body and overall well-being.

Incorporating fresh juices made from fruits, vegetables, and leafy greens into your daily routine is an excellent practice for maintaining a healthy and energetic body. With endless combinations to explore, you can enjoy not only flavorful and refreshing options but also targeted health benefits, such as relief from conditions like arthritis, thanks to essential nutrients that support wellness. Making this a part of your everyday life can transform your health, boost your energy, and elevate your quality of life. Try it for yourself and feel the difference!

Juices: Unleash Their Power

Incorporating smoothies or shakes into your diet can be an excellent way to enhance your health. Here are some of their most notable benefits:

▸ **Compliance with Recommended Fruit and Vegetable Intake**: Smoothies and shakes offer a practical and enjoyable way to meet the daily recommendation of five servings of fruits and vegetables. They provide a diverse range of essential nutrients that support optimal health and overall well-being.

‣ **Easy Assimilation and Digestion**: As liquid meals, smoothies and shakes are gentler on the digestive system and allow for quicker nutrient absorption. They are especially beneficial for individuals with digestive sensitivities or challenges.

‣ **Vitamin and Mineral Powerhouse**: Made from fresh fruits and vegetables, smoothies and shakes are rich sources of essential vitamins and minerals that promote the proper functioning of the body.

‣ **Detoxification and Cleansing**: Ingredients like leafy greens and natural antioxidants help flush out toxins, enhance cell health, and support effective internal cleansing.

‣ **Balancing Body pH**: By incorporating alkaline foods, smoothies and shakes play a key role in stabilizing the body's pH levels, aiding disease prevention and improving overall wellness.

‣ **Reduction of Inflammation**: Anti-inflammatory additions such as turmeric, ginger, and leafy greens can help minimize inflammation, fostering better health and increased comfort.

‣ **A Balanced Meal Replacement**: When combined with protein, healthy fats, and complex carbohydrates, smoothies become a nourishing and balanced meal replacement. They provide sustained energy and promote fullness throughout the day.

‣ **Supports Weight Management**: With their low-calorie yet nutrient-dense profiles, smoothies and shakes encourage healthy eating habits. They help manage appetite and support maintaining or achieving an ideal weight.

‣ **Enhances Skin Health**: Packed with skin-friendly vitamins like A and C from fresh ingredients, smoothies and shakes contribute to hydrated, radiant, and healthy skin.

‣ **Slows Cellular Aging**: The antioxidants in smoothie ingredients combat oxidative damage, protect cells, and help maintain a youthful appearance.

▸ **Boosts Energy and Vitality**: Smoothies made with superfoods provide a steady energy boost, helping you stay active, energized, and revitalized throughout the day.

In conclusion, smoothies and shakes are a nutritious, convenient, and versatile addition to your diet. Not only do they make it easier to meet your daily fruit and vegetable intake, but they also offer a wide array of health benefits. Packed with essential nutrients, they support overall well-being–all while being refreshing, delicious, and easy to enjoy.

Homemade vs. Commercial Juices

Nowadays, identifying which foods truly benefit our health can be quite challenging. Supermarkets are overflowing with an extensive range of options, flaunting attractive packaging and clever designs that promise to be natural and healthy. While advertising and packaging often catch our attention, are we genuinely purchasing natural beverages made from fruits and vegetables? Do you know the key differences between homemade juices and industrial products? Are packaged products really as nutritious as they claim to be? Taking a few moments to carefully read ingredient labels and analyze their composition may uncover some surprising truths.

A few years ago, international regulations were established to define the standards that every fruit-based beverage must meet, specifying precise characteristics for each type of product. Below, we'll explore these distinctions and delve into the essential differences.

▸ **Fruit Juice**

Fruit juice is derived from fresh, chilled, or frozen fruits without undergoing any fermentation. It may contain separately extracted pulp and, in some cases, be blended with juice from various fruits. Labels are required to specify the composition in descending order, including the exact percentage of each fruit.

To prolong shelf life and eliminate the need for refrigeration, fruit juice is typically sterilized or pasteurized. Unfortunately, these processes result in significant nutrient loss, particularly impacting essential vitamins and enzymes. Moreover, the juice lacks the natural fiber found in whole fruits.

▸ Juice from Concentrates

Juice from concentrates is created by reconstituting dehydrated juice concentrates with water. Concentrates are produced by extracting natural juice through evaporation or other physical methods. During reconstitution, manufacturers may add aromas or pulp from similar fruits to partially restore flavor.

Though widely consumed, these juices suffer nutrient losses during production, including enzymes, vitamins, minerals, and the valuable fiber that characterizes natural fruit.

▸ Dehydrated or Powdered Fruit Juice

This product is manufactured by removing water from fruit to create a dry powder, which can later be rehydrated or sold in its dehydrated state. However, the dehydration process significantly diminishes its nutritional value, leading to the loss of enzymes, vitamins, minerals, and natural fiber.

▸ Fruit Nectar

Fruit nectar differs from pure juice as it is made using fruit concentrate, water, and added sugars or sweeteners. Its nutritional value is considerably lower compared to natural fruit juices due to its inclusion of artificial additives to enhance flavor, color, or shelf life.

▸ Juice-Based Drinks

These beverages typically combine various fruits but contain minimal actual fruit juice. Often, they lack the essential nutrients derived from fruits, consisting largely of water, artificial aromas, colorings, and sweeteners.

▸ Milk-Infused Juice Drinks

Milk-infused juice drinks include fruit juice, often from concentrates, in very small proportions. They are mixed with milk, water, flavorings, and other ingredients. These beverages are not considered true juices, and any nutrients present are artificially added during manufacturing to compensate for losses incurred during processing.

‣ **Vegetable and/or Greens Juice**
Vegetable and greens juices are extracted from vegetables using specialized industrial methods, often with added pulp or pureed ingredients. They may also blend various vegetables to create balanced or palatable flavors.

To extend shelf life and eliminate refrigeration requirements, these juices undergo pasteurization or sterilization, which unfortunately reduces essential nutrients, including vitamins and phytonutrients. Additionally, they lack the natural fiber of whole vegetables and may include preservatives, salt, or flavor enhancers that compromise their nutritional profile.

‣ **Commercial Smoothies**
Commercial smoothies are typically prepared by blending fruits, vegetables, and greens–often using purees or concentrates–with water, milk, plant-based beverages, or similar liquids. Their thicker texture comes from a higher proportion of pulp or fiber-rich components.

To enhance taste, appearance, and shelf life, industrial smoothies usually contain added sugars, preservatives, colorings, and flavorings that alter their natural composition. Moreover, they undergo pasteurization or thermal sterilization to allow room-temperature storage, further degrading their original nutrients and reducing their overall nutritional quality.

Advantages of Homemade Juices

After discovering what commercial products truly contain, it becomes evident that making juices at home offers numerous advantages. Here are the key benefits:

‣ **Complete Control Over Ingredients**: Preparing your own juices allows you to ensure the quality of the ingredients you use. There are no unnecessary additives, no preservatives, and –most importantly–no unpleasant surprises.

‣ **Variety and Creativity**: You have the freedom to choose your favorite fruits and vegetables, experiment with unique combinations, or incorporate fresh, seasonal produce. This not only provides a burst of delicious flavors but also boosts your intake of essential nutrients.

▸ **Authentic Aroma and Flavor**: Homemade juices retain the genuine aroma and taste of fresh fruits and vegetables. There's truly nothing like enjoying a freshly made juice packed with natural freshness.

▸ **Maximum Nutrient Retention**: Vitamins, minerals, antioxidants, enzymes, and other nutrients remain intact when you prepare juices at home, significantly enhancing their health benefits.

▸ **Premium Quality Ingredients**: Choosing fresh, seasonal produce at its peak ripeness ensures optimal flavor and exceptional nutritional value.

▸ **Seasonal Food Benefits**: Consuming fruits and vegetables that are in season supports sustainability, is more cost-effective, and often results in better taste and nutritional quality.

▸ **Total Customization**: Whether using a juicer or blender, you can adjust the consistency of your juice to your liking–whether you prefer a light, clear juice or a thicker, fiber-rich option.

▸ **Kid-Friendly Option**: Homemade juices are an excellent way to incorporate fruits and vegetables into children's diets, especially for picky eaters. With creative flavors and fun presentations, you can make juices irresistible for kids.

Making juices at home provides several compelling advantages: complete control over ingredients, enhanced nutrient retention, and the flexibility to tailor your drinks to your preferences. It's also a simple yet effective way to promote healthy eating for the whole family.

Possible Adverse Effects

If you suffer from **gastritis, colitis, SIBO, irritable bowel syndrome, or constipation**, it's essential to take certain precautions when preparing smoothies or juices. Following these recommendations will help you enjoy their benefits without worsening your symptoms:

▸ **Use a juicer instead of a blender**: For digestive health conditions, it's often better to use a juicer rather than a blender when making juices. Juicing removes most of the fiber from the ingredients, resulting in a smoother liquid that is gentler on your digestive system.

▸ **Moderate your fiber intake**: Although fiber is highly beneficial for overall health, excessive consumption can lead to gas, bloating, or constipation–especially for individuals with sensitive digestion. Be mindful of the fiber content in your smoothies by limiting ingredients like fruit pulp, seeds, and whole grains.

▸ **Introduce juices gradually**: If you're unsure how your body will react, start with small portions. This enables you to monitor their effects on your digestion and adjust the recipes to suit your specific needs.

▸ **Consume juices on an empty stomach**: Drinking juices on an empty stomach can maximize nutrient absorption and aid digestion. This approach minimizes the risk of digestive discomfort and helps you fully benefit from the juice's nutrients.

▸ **Tailor recipes to your personal needs**: Everyone's digestive system is unique, and responses to certain foods can vary greatly. Pay close attention to how your body reacts after consuming juices, and adapt ingredient combinations to best support your health and well-being.

When to Take Them

There are several effective ways to incorporate juices into your routine, depending on your goals and daily habits. Below are three recommended methods:

▸ **In the morning, on an empty stomach**: Begin your day with a carefully chosen juice recipe, consuming it before eating anything else. Drinking juice on an empty stomach enhances nutrient absorption and stimulates your digestive system, helping prepare it for the rest of the day.

▸ **On an empty stomach, before meals**: Enjoy a juice approximately 30 minutes before your main meals to maximize its benefits. This practice supports digestion and boosts nutrient absorption, promoting overall health and well-being.

▸ **Juice-based fasting**: Engage in a multi-day fast consisting exclusively of juices to achieve specific health objectives or to detoxify your body. Choose 2 to 3 recipes and consume them consistently throughout the day to stay nourished and energized.

Preparation Tips

Preparing fresh juices is an easy and nutritious way to make the most of the vitamins and minerals found in fruits and vegetables. To optimize the process and ensure safety, consider the following recommendations:

▸ **Choose organic ingredients**: Whenever possible, opt for organic fruits and vegetables. They provide cleaner, pesticide-free consumption and promote a healthier lifestyle.

▸ **Wash ingredients thoroughly**: Rinse all produce carefully to remove dirt, bacteria, and chemical residues. Trim any bruised, moldy, or damaged areas to prevent contamination.

▸ **Cut ingredients into smaller pieces**: Make blending easier by chopping fruits and vegetables into smaller, manageable chunks. This helps achieve a smoother texture and shortens preparation time.

▸ **Balance ingredients with low water content**: Fruits and vegetables with low water content, such as bananas and avocados, may require pre-mixing. Start with juicier ingredients to create a liquid base, then gradually add denser items for a cohesive blend.

‣ **Peel certain fruits appropriately**: Remove citrus rinds (like those from oranges and grapefruits), as their outer layers may contain toxins. However, keep the nutrient-rich white inner layer. Peel tropical fruits, such as papayas and kiwis, especially if they are grown in regions with less stringent chemical regulations.

‣ **Discard harmful seeds**: Remove seeds from apples, as they contain trace amounts of cyanide and are unsafe to consume. On the other hand, seeds from grapes, melons, lemons, and limes are safe and offer additional health benefits.

‣ **Incorporate stems and leaves mindfully**: Many stems and leaves are nutritious, but be cautious. Avoid toxic ones, such as carrot and rhubarb leaves, which can be harmful.

‣ **Drink your juice immediately**: Freshly prepared juice is best consumed right away to minimize nutrient loss and avoid oxidation. This ensures maximum freshness and health benefits.

‣ **Remove bitter celery leaves**: Bitter celery leaves can affect the flavor of your juice. Remove them before blending the stalks to create a more balanced and enjoyable taste.

Key Recommendations

Smoothies and shakes are an excellent, healthy alternative, but to get the most out of them, it's essential to keep certain aspects in mind. Below are some key recommendations:

‣ **Moderate fruit consumption**: Fruits are a fantastic source of nutrients but also contain fructose, a natural sugar that, when consumed excessively, can impact your health. Strive for balance by moderating your fruit intake throughout the day. Additionally, avoid eating fruits at night, as the body may metabolize them less efficiently during this time.

‣ **Choose seasonal fruits**: Seasonal fruits are often more nutrient-rich, flavorful, and cost-effective. By opting for fruits in season, you can enjoy their peak freshness and nutritional benefits while saving money.

▸ **Pick compatible combinations**: Not all fruits or ingredients blend well together. Research suitable pairings to create a smoothie or shake with balanced flavors and optimal nutritional value.

▸ **Use a moderate amount of ingredients**: The simplest smoothies are often the best. Avoid overloading them with excessive ingredients, which can lead to heavy textures or digestive discomfort. Stick to recommended recipes and be mindful of proportions.

▸ **Include leafy greens and vegetables**: Incorporate leafy greens, like spinach or kale, or vegetables, such as cucumber, to lower the glycemic index and boost your drink's nutrient profile. These additions make your smoothie both healthier and more satisfying.

▸ **Use natural sweeteners in moderation**: Enjoy the natural flavors of the ingredients, but if sweetening is necessary, choose options like raw honey or pure stevia. Use them sparingly to maintain a balanced nutritional profile.

▸ **Chew your drink**: Even liquid smoothies benefit from being "chewed." This simple habit stimulates the release of digestive enzymes, helping improve nutrient absorption and reducing discomfort like bloating or indigestion.

▸ **Store properly**: For the best results, consume smoothies or shakes fresh. If storing is needed, place them in a dark, airtight container in the refrigerator, or freeze individual portions for later use.

▸ **Make them fun and personalized**: Add an enjoyable twist by freezing smoothies in molds with fun shapes–an excellent way to turn a healthy drink into a delightful treat, especially for children.

These recommendations will help you make the most of your smoothies and shakes. While the recipes provided in this book are crafted to facilitate nutrient absorption, always remember that individual needs vary. Feel free to experiment with different combinations, tailor recipes to suit your tastes, and prioritize your health and well-being. Enjoy the journey to a healthier lifestyle!

Nutritious Juice Recipes for Gastritis

▸ **Carrot, beet and cucumber juice**

Ingredients: 2 or 3 carrots, 1/2 cucumber, 1/2 beet with leaves. Preparation: cut the carrots into strips of 5 to 7 cm. Cut the cucumber into several pieces and then into strips. Cut the beet into thin slices. Pass it all through the blender (also effective for reflux or acidity).

▸ **Carrot and spinach juice**

Ingredients: 6 to 7 carrots and a bunch of spinach. Preparation: Clean the carrots and cut them into 5 to 7-centimeter-long strips. Blend the ingredients, starting and ending with the carrot (this method is also effective for reflux or acidity).

▸ **Carrot, cabbage and celery or red cabbage juice**

Ingredients: 2 carrots, 4 celery sticks, and 1 slice (8 cm) of red cabbage. Preparation: Cut the carrots into 5–to 7-cm-long strips. Cut the celery in the same way. Then, cut the cabbage into thin slices. Blend everything.

▸ **Beet, broccoli and carrot juice**

Ingredients: 100 grams of beet, 100 grams of broccoli, and 150 grams of carrot. Preparation: cut the beet and carrot into pieces. Cut the broccoli flowers and discard the stalks. Blend the ingredients.

▸ **Fennel and apple juice**

Ingredients: 120 grams of fennel (1 small bulb or half of a large one) and 3 apples. Preparation: cut the fennel and the apple into thin slices. Pass them through the blender.

▸ **Carrot and cucumber juice**

Ingredients: 4 carrots and 1/2 cucumber. Pass it all through the blender.

Carrot and leek juice: Four carrots and half a tender leek are the ingredients. Wash and blend them to prepare them.

▸ **Potato, carrot, apple and parsley juice**
Ingredients: 1 potato slice, 4 carrots, 1 apple, and a handful of parsley. Slice the potato into thin slices. Slice the carrots into 5- to 7-cm-long strips. Slice the apple into thin slices. Blend all the ingredients (this method is also effective for reflux or heartburn).

▸ **Carrot, apple, and ginger juice**
Ingredients: 200 grams of carrot, 1 apple, and 1/2 tablespoon of ginger. Preparation: Cut the carrot and apple into quarters. Finely chop the ginger. Blend the ingredients and strain to remove the hard ginger.

▸ **Fennel, beet, and apple juice**
Ingredients: 180 g fennel (1 medium bulb), 1/4 beet with leaves, and 2 apples. To prepare, cut all the ingredients into thin slices and blend them.

▸ **Carrot juice, sweet turnip and parsley**
Ingredients: 6 or 7 carrots, 1 slice of sweet turnip, 2 and a half centimeters long, and a handful of parsley. Preparation: Cut the turnips into strips. Clean the carrots and cut them into strips 5 to 7 centimeters long. Blend the ingredients.

▸ **Carrot, potato, watercress and parsley juice**
Ingredients: 5 carrots, 1/4 potato, 4 watercress, and 4 parsley sprigs. Preparation: Clean the carrots and cut them into 5 to 7 cm strips. Cut the potato into thin slices. Pass all the ingredients through the blender (effective for reflux or acidity).

▸ **Papaya and grapefruit juice**
Ingredients: 1 papaya and 2 grapefruits. Preparation: peel the papaya, remove the seeds, and chop it. Peel the grapefruit, remove the white part, and cut into pieces. Blend ingredients.

▸ **Apple, carrot, and beet juice**
Ingredients: 1 apple, 1/2 carrot, 1 beet, and 100 ml water. Preparation: cut the apple and beet into quarters and the carrot

into slices. Blend it all. Pour into a glass and add the water.

▸ Carrot, cabbage, and celery juice

Ingredients: 2 carrots, 1/4 cabbage, and 1 celery stalk. Preparation: cut the carrots and celery into strips and the cabbage into slices. Pass it all through the blender. Take 3 times a day (effective also for reflux or heartburn).

▸ Cabbage, celery, broccoli and parsley juice

Ingredients: 1/4 cup cabbage, 2 celery stalks, 1 broccoli sprig and 1 parsley leaf. To prepare, blend all the ingredients (this is also effective for reflux or acidity).

▸ Cucumber juice with lemon* and grapefruit

Ingredients: 350 g cucumber, 1/4 lemon*, and 1/2 grapefruit. Preparation: Chop the cucumber, peel the lemon* and grapefruit, remove the white part, and chop them. Blend all the ingredients. Pour the mixture into a pitcher, adding water if it seems too strong.

(*Refer to the chapter "Foods That Transform", section "Lemon and Gastritis: Myth or Remedy?" for more information).

MEDICINAL PLANTS

Since time immemorial, humanity has turned to the natural world for answers to its needs. Medicinal herbs, faithful companions on this journey, have generously shared their wisdom to ease ailments and enhance well-being. This ancient knowledge, carefully preserved through the ages, has found a renewed place in the modern world, offering a healthy and sustainable option to address today's challenges.

In a society increasingly conscious of the adverse effects of certain pharmaceutical treatments and the environmental toll of unsustainable practices, botanical remedies are experiencing a resurgence with renewed prominence. For those seeking a balanced, respectful lifestyle in harmony with the environ-ment, these green treasures provide invaluable solutions. This revival not only reflects a growing interest in ecological approaches but also an evolution toward holistic care for both the body and the planet.

What makes these natural wonders truly extraordinary is the complexity of their compounds, capable of delivering anti-inflammatory, antioxidant, antibacterial, and antiviral proper-ties, among others. Their potential ranges from alleviating everyday issues like sleeplessness or sluggish digestion to addressing conditions such as chronic stress or age-related ailments.

Beyond the ability to target specific concerns, these species serve as vital sources of micronutrients–vitamins, minerals, fiber, and antioxidants–that fortify the immune system and support long-term health. Incorporating them into dietary or self-care routines offers a simple, sustainable, and effective path toward illness prevention and enhanced overall wellness.

The botanical kingdom boasts remarkable diversity, featuring countless species uniquely suited to meet specific needs. Whether prepared as herbal teas, applied as balms or tinctures, or utilized in the form of essential oils, their applications are as versatile as they are effective, seamlessly fitting into various lifestyles.

More than mere remedies, these natural allies inspire us to reconnect with the world around us. Harnessing their benefits requires respect for environmental rhythms and a deeper appreciation for our planet's ecosystems. Each herb or extract serves as a tangible reminder of our connection to the living world, fostering a sense of harmony that transcends the physical and nurtures the spiritual.

In addition to their myriad health benefits, plant-based solutions stand out for their accessibility and practical versatility. Many species grow abundantly in wild habitats or can be easily cultivated in home gardens, offering an affordable, sustainable alternative. In a global context marked by economic inequalities, these wellness allies provide inclusive options to complement—or even replace—costly interventions.

Over the centuries, knowledge of these natural solutions has been carefully preserved through oral traditions and written records. This heritage, rooted in deep respect for biodiversity, has been bolstered by modern science, validating the effects of their active compounds and shedding light on their mechanisms of action. It represents a powerful synergy between tradition and innovation, broadening the therapeutic applications of these botanical marvels.

However, unlocking their full potential requires responsible use. Every human body is unique, and while these species possess well-documented therapeutic properties, they are not without risks. Misuse or interactions with conventional medications can lead to adverse effects. Therefore, obtaining accurate and reliable information is essential to ensure safe and effective usage.

One particularly fascinating aspect is how the components

within a plant work in unison. Whole extracts, resulting from this intricate interaction, often produce more balanced and holistic effects compared to isolated compounds. Molecules interact in complementary ways, maximizing benefits while reducing potential side effects. Conversely, isolated active principles can provide concentrated solutions but may carry an increased risk of adverse effects on the body.

The innate harmony of these botanical wonders highlights one of biodiversity's greatest gifts–balance. Whole extracts are celebrated for their gentleness and ability to integrate seamlessly with the body's natural processes. On the other hand, synthesized compounds strive for potency, often at the expense of stability. The synergistic interaction between molecular components amplifies therapeutic benefits while limiting potential downsides, making them a choice deeply aligned with human needs.

Ultimately, medicinal plants transcend their role as therapeutic tools–they bridge ancestral wisdom and scientific innovation. They remind us that the health of our bodies and the well-being of our planet are profoundly interconnected. By safeguarding this invaluable legacy, we nurture not only our own health but also that of future generations, renewing the delicate balance between humanity and nature.

Essential Information

Although plants are natural in origin, they should not be considered entirely harmless. Their active compounds may cause adverse effects or trigger allergies in certain individuals.

Occasional consumption of an infusion is unlikely to cause harm. However, excessive, prolonged, or frequent use may result in discomfort, allergic reactions, or even toxicity.

Tolerance to natural remedies varies greatly among people. If you are pregnant, breastfeeding, or managing conditions such as chronic illnesses, allergies, kidney or liver insufficiency, cancer, or undergoing medical treatment, it is crucial to refer to the section titled **"Learn Everything You Need to Know About the Plants"** before using them. This section provides essential information on potential risks, contraindications, and interactions, enabling you to make informed and responsible decisions.

Guidelines for Care with Herbal Remedies

For best results, continue using the remedies until your symptoms have completely disappeared. The treatment duration will vary depending on factors like the severity of your condition, how it progresses, your personal commitment, and other important influences.

Keep in mind that some plants or herbal remedies are not suited for continuous or long-term use. In such cases, you will always find specific instructions that address this.

While following the guidelines for the remedies below, it is just as important to focus on the underlying causes of your symptoms. To better understand the root of your health concerns, I recommend referring to the first chapter of this book, specifically the section titled "Causes", where you'll discover essential insights into tackling the problem at its source.

Finally, remember that patience is vital. A condition that has lingered for months or years cannot be resolved in just a few days. Stay committed, persevere, and always prioritize your health and well-being.

Medicinal Plants for Gastritis

Nature offers us numerous allies to help relieve the symptoms of gastritis, with some of the most effective options being **aloe vera, green anise, boldo, fennel, ginger, chamomile, licorice, and rosemary**. These medicinal plants are renowned for their soothing and digestive properties, assisting in reducing pain and other symptoms associated with this condition.

It is advisable to select one or two of these plants and consume them for a period of three weeks. After this time, switch to other plants for the same duration, and continue alternating in this manner until noticeable improvement occurs. This method ensures a balanced use of each plant's benefits without overloading the body with a single one.

The ideal way to consume these plants is by preparing natural infusions or decoctions, as sweeteners can harm the stomach lining. If sweetening is absolutely necessary, the best option is 100% natural stevia, which is gentler on the digestive system.

It is crucial to pay attention to the preparation and dosage of these plants to maximize their benefits. Including their scientific names in parentheses can help with accurate identification, as common names might vary depending on the region or country.

Aloe vera (Aloe barbadensis)

Aloe gel effectively reduces stomach and esophagus irritations, regenerating and protecting its walls. It also reduces and even completely relieves inflammation and heals wounds caused by gastric or duodenal ulcers. It helps reduce inflammation in cases of gastritis and duodenitis, stimulates digestion, reduces stomach acidity, and restores the internal pH of the stomach. It is also effective in treating infectious stomach diseases. Here are some remedies:

Take 1 tablespoon of aloe vera gel about 15-20 minutes before each main meal. If you do not like its taste, you can mix it with some natural juice or infusion.

You can also take 2 tablespoons of aloe vera gel with a pinch of baking soda to experience immediate relief. (Note: Avoid excessive use of baking soda due to its high salt content, as it can cause adverse effects such as nausea and bloating, among others).

In tablets or drops, take 3 times a day without exceeding the daily dose of 0.5 grams.

Note: If you also suffer from reflux, aloe vera is one of the most effective plants for treating it.

Boldo (Peumus boldus)

Infusion: Use 2 teaspoons of dried boldo leaves and 1 liter of water. Boil the water in a saucepan, and before it boils, add the boldo. Let it cook for 3 minutes, then remove it from the heat. Cover and let stand for another 2 minutes; strain and drink. The recommended dose is 1 cup, 2 or 3 times a day.

Chamomile (Chamaemelum nobile)

Chamomile improves digestion and promotes relaxation. By facilitating digestion, it decreases the risk of reflux and neutralizes the acidic pH of the stomach. In addition, it repairs and protects the gastric membrane. It also helps expel intestinal gas, relieve stomach pains, prevent nausea or vomiting, and help treat colic, gastritis and gastric ulcers. Recipe:

Infusion: Use 1 teaspoon of dried chamomile flowers and honey (optional). Boil 1 cup of water in a saucepan, reduce the heat, add chamomile, and simmer for 1 minute. Remove from heat and let steep for 2 more minutes. Pour the infusion into a cup and add a little honey. Drink this infusion after eating and half an hour before bed.

Fennel (Foeniculum vulgare)

Infusion: Crush the fennel seeds and use 1 tablespoon per cup of water. Boil the water and then remove it from the heat. Add the crushed fennel seeds, cover them, and steep them for 10 minutes. Strain and drink 1 cup per day.

Ginger (Zingiber officinale)

Ginger contains phenols that help relieve irritation. It is anti-inflammatory and facilitates digestion, improving both gastritis and reflux. It is also used to fight Helicobacter Pylori bacteria, which causes some stomach ulcers. In addition, it helps to eliminate accumulated gases and fight abdominal distension. Here are some remedies:

Infusion: Combine 1-2 grams of peeled ginger and 1 cup of water. Boil the water and ginger for 5-10 minutes. Strain and drink 2 times a day.

Decoction: Use 1 or 2 grams of chopped ginger root, a little lemon*, and 500 ml water. Heat the water, and when it boils, add the ginger pieces to lower the heat. Cover and let it cook for about 15 to 20 minutes. Please turn off the heat and let it stand for 5 more minutes. Strain and add a few drops of lemon*, as the flavor of this infusion is strong. Drink 1 or 2 times a day.

Capsules: Take 1 to 2 grams per day.
Dried or fresh ginger: Add chopped or grated ginger to the food.

See "Lemon and Gastritis: Myth or Remedy?", in the Chapter "Foods That Transform" for more information.

Green Anise (Pimpinella anisum)

Decoction: Use 1 tablespoon of green anise and 750 ml of water (3 glasses). Boil the water in a saucepan and add the anise. Boil for 5 minutes, then turn off the heat, remove the anise, and let it stand for 10 minutes. Filter the liquid and drink it three times daily, before or after meals.

Infusion: Crush the anise seeds and use 1 teaspoon of coffee per cup of water. Boil the water and add the crushed anise seeds. Cover and let it steep for 10 minutes. Strain the liquid and drink it neat or sweetened with stevia. Drink it two or three times a day, before or after meals.

Licorice (Glycyrrhiza glabra)

This root has soothing properties for the stomach, as it is anti-inflammatory, antispasmodic, and antacid. It also prevents stomach heaviness, reduces gas, and prevents indigestion. Remedies:

Decoction: Use 1 teaspoon of dried root and 1 glass of water. Heat the water, and when it starts to boil, add the licorice and let it cook for 10 minutes. Remove from heat and let stand for 10-15 minutes. Sweeten with stevia. Drink 2 or 3 cups a day.

Infusion: Use 1-2 teaspoons of grated licorice root. Let the licorice soak in a bowl of cold water for 12 hours. Drink a cup every day for 3-4 weeks.

Chew a small amount of licorice, but do not swallow it immediately. If the licorice is in pill form, let it dissolve in your mouth without chewing. This will allow it to mix well with saliva, which is better.

Chew 3 licorice wafers without glycerin 2 or 3 times a day.
Note: It is better to use licorice without glycyrrhizin, often called "DGL licorice", as this component has some contra-indications.

Rosemary (Rosmarinus officinalis)

Infusion: Use 1 tablespoon of rosemary leaves per 750 ml of water (3 glasses). Heat the water over the fire and bring it to a boil. Remove the water from the heat, add the rosemary, cover it, and let it steep for 15-20 minutes. Strain and drink alone or sweetened with stevia. Drink three times a day, before or after meals.

Decoction: Use 1 or 2 teaspoons of dried rosemary herb per cup of water. Bring the water to a boil. When it starts to boil, add the rosemary and let it cook for 3 more minutes. Please turn off the heat, cover, and let it steep for 8 minutes. Strain and sweeten with stevia. Drink 2 or 3 cups a day, before or after meals

Phytotherapy Recipes

Although the plants mentioned above are effective when used individually, their properties can be further enhanced when combined properly. Below are some particularly effective combinations.

› **Phytotherapy recipe nº 1**

Ingredients: boldo, lemon balm, chamomile, green anise, mallow and marshmallow.

Preparation: Mix the plants in equal parts. Add 4 table-spoons of the mixture to 1 liter of water. Put the mixture on the fire, and when it starts to boil, reduce the heat and cover it for 5 minutes. Please remove it from the heat and let it stand for 10 more minutes. Then, divide the preparation into 6 cups. After digestion, consume 1 cup after each meal (breakfast, lunch and dinner) and 3 cups between meals. You can drink it unsweetened or with stevia.

> **Phytotherapy Recipe No. 2**

Ingredients: 1/2 teaspoon of fennel seeds, 1/2 teaspoon of green anise, 1/2 teaspoon of chamomile flowers, and 1 cup of water.

Preparation: Heat the water and add the anise and fennel when it boils. Let it cook for 3 minutes, then remove it from the heat. Add the chamomile, cover it, and steep it for 5 minutes. You can drink it alone or sweeten it with stevia. Take it two or three times a day after meals.

> **Phytotherapy recipe nº 3**

Ingredients: yarrow (30%), lemon balm (25%), rosemary (15%), calendula (15%), and marjoram (15%).

Preparation: Mix all the herbs. Add 3 to 4 tablespoons of the mixture to every half-liter of water. Put the mix of plants in the water and bring it to a boil for 1 minute. Please turn off the heat, cover, and let it stand for 10 minutes. Drink three times a day, half an hour before meals. It is not necessary to sweeten it.

Note: This recipe also effectively treats stomach nerves, gastric or gastroduodenal ulcers and gastric acidity.

Learn Everything You Need to Know About the Plants

In this section, we'll delve into the most recommended botanical species for treating the condition at hand. You'll find essential information about their possible adverse effects, contraindications, and interactions, as well as detailed insights into each plant. From their descriptions and habitats to their uses, chemical components, histories, and therapeutic properties, this chapter is designed to take you on a fascinating journey of discovery.

My goal is to provide you with a comprehensive understanding of these plants, helping you grasp their context and fully appreciate their many benefits. We'll explore their historical origins and significance in traditional medicine, highlighting their invaluable role in natural care.

I want you to become an expert on these species, capable of making informed decisions in your pursuit of wellness. Get ready to expand your knowledge and uncover the extraordinary healing power of nature!

Aloe vera (Aloe barbadensis)

Description:
Aloe vera, also known as aloe vera, is a perennial succulent plant in the lily family. Its leaves are fleshy and lanceolate and grow in a rosette.

Habitat and cultivation:
This plant thrives in warm, dry climates, preferably with temperatures between 20 and 30 degrees Celsius. It requires well-drained soil and does not tolerate excess moisture. It reproduces by leaf cuttings and can be grown in pots or gardens.

Parts used:
The main parts of Aloe vera used are the leaves, which contain a transparent gel inside. These are obtained by cutting and opening the fresh leaves. The dried leaves and the yellow sap under the leaves' skin are also occasionally used.

Components:
Aloe vera gel contains polysaccharides, vitamins (such as C and E), minerals (such as calcium, magnesium and zinc), enzymes, amino acids and antioxidants, all contributing to its therapeutic properties.

History and tradition:
Aloe vera has a long history of use. It was known as "the plant of immortality" in ancient Egypt. It has also been used in traditional Chinese and Ayurvedic medicine. Over the centuries, its reputation as a medicinal plant has spread worldwide.

Therapeutic properties:
Aloe vera juice treats burns, wounds, insect bites, and skin

conditions such as psoriasis and acne. It has also been used to relieve skin irritation and inflammation. Consumption of Aloe vera juice is associated with digestive health benefits, relieving constipation and promoting intestinal health.

Curiosities:

Aloe vera has some interesting curiosities associated with its history and use. For example, it is believed that Cleopatra used Aloe vera gel as part of her beauty routine. In World War II, Aloe vera gel was used as a blood substitute in emergencies, as its chemical composition resembled that of blood plasma. It has also been used in the food industry as an additive in yogurts and beverages.

Adverse or side effects:

Although Aloe vera is generally safe for topical use and moderate oral consumption, some individuals may experience adverse effects. Some people may have allergic reactions or skin irritation when applying Aloe vera gel. In rare cases, excessive consumption of Aloe vera juice may cause diarrhea, abdominal cramps and electrolyte imbalances. In addition, it has been reported that prolonged use of high concentrations of Aloe vera on the skin may cause dryness and flaking.

Contraindications:

Although Aloe vera is considered safe for most people, some contraindications exist. It is not recommended for topical use on deep wounds, severe burns, or open surgical wounds, as it may delay healing. In addition, pregnant and nursing women should consult a healthcare professional before using Aloe vera products, as there may be potential risks to the fetus or baby.

Interactions:

Aloe can interact with certain medications and supplements, so it is essential to exercise caution when combined with other products. For example, Aloe vera may increase the risk of bleeding in people taking anticoagulants such as warfarin. It has also been reported that Aloe vera may interfere with the absorption of oral medications, such as angiotensin-converting enzyme inhibitors (ACE inhibitors) used to treat high blood pressure.

Boldo (Peumus boldus)

Description:
Boldo is a perennial shrub in the Monimiaceae family. It is native to South America, specifically Chile, and has spread to other regions with similar climates. Boldo has leathery, lanceolate, dark green leaves. Its flowers are small and yellow; when ripe, it produces small, round black fruits. Its strong aroma and bitter taste characterize Boldo.

Habitat and cultivation:
Boldo grows wild in mountainous areas with Mediterranean and subtropical climates. It requires well-drained soils and prefers areas with sun exposure. As for its cultivation, it can be propagated through seeds, although it is also common to reproduce it by cuttings. It is a hardy plant and can tolerate drought conditions.

Parts used:
The parts used are mainly the leaves. These are harvested manually and dried for later use. The dried leaves contain the beneficial compounds that give the plant medicinal properties.

Components:
Boldo contains several chemical constituents that give it its therapeutic properties. Some main components include alkaloids (such as boldine), flavonoids, essential oils, tannins and antioxidant compounds. These compounds contribute to the medicinal properties of boldo.

History and tradition:
Boldo has a long history of use in traditional South American medicine. The indigenous peoples of Chile used it to treat various digestive disorders, such as indigestion and colic. In some cultures, it is also considered a sacred plant and has been used in rituals and ceremonies to purify the body and spirit.

Therapeutic properties:
Boldo is primarily used for its digestive and liver-supporting properties. Some of its therapeutic benefits include stimulating

bile production and aiding in the digestion of fats. It can alleviate digestive issues such as indigestion, stomach upset, and gas. Additionally, Boldo helps protect and enhance liver function, assisting in the body's detoxification. It also possesses antioxidant and anti-inflammatory properties. Traditionally, it is used as a mild diuretic to relieve symptoms of cystitis.

Curiosities:
Boldo is a plant highly valued in traditional medicine throughout South America. It is also used to make beverages and liquors, such as the famous "pisco sour" in Chile. In Argentina and Chile, boldo is a national symbol of healing and protective properties. In popular tradition, it is believed to help relieve hangovers and soothe stomach upset caused by excessive alcohol consumption.

Adverse or side effects:
Boldo is generally considered safe when consumed in moderate amounts. However, some people may experience side effects, such as stomach upset, nausea, vomiting, or diarrhea. Consuming it in excessive quantities may irritate the stomach and kidneys, and in extreme cases, it could lead to liver damage. Additionally, some people may be allergic to boldo, so caution is advised for those with known sensitivities to plants in the Monimiaceae family.

Contraindications:
It is not recommended for pregnant or breastfeeding women to use Boldo, as it may stimulate uterine activity, and there is not enough evidence to confirm its safety in these situations. Additionally, individuals with severe liver or kidney disease should avoid taking Boldo, as it could worsen these conditions. People with bile duct obstruction or gallstones should also refrain from using it, as it may exacerbate symptoms or lead to complications.

Interactions:
Boldo may interact with certain medications, including anticoagulants and antiplatelet drugs, which can increase the risk of bleeding. Therefore, exercising caution is essential; you should consult a physician if you take these medications.

Additionally, due to its diuretic effect, boldo may enhance the effects of diuretic drugs, potentially leading to increased fluid and electrolyte loss. If you're on medications that are metabolized by the liver, such as specific cholesterol medications or oral contraceptives, boldo may interfere with their metabolism and reduce their effectiveness.

Calendula (Calendula officinalis)

Description:
Calendula is an annual or biennial herbaceous plant belonging to the Asteraceae family. It is characterized by light green, lanceolate leaves and large, showy flowers, usually bright yellow or orange. Marigold flowers resemble daisies, with reed-shaped petals and a center filled with small tubular flowers.

Habitat and cultivation:
Marigold is native to the Mediterranean region but has naturalized in many parts of the world. It prefers to grow in temperate, sunny climates, although it can tolerate partial shade. It adapts well to different types of well-drained soils and is commonly found in gardens, fields and meadows.

As for cultivation, marigolds can be grown from seeds sown in spring or autumn. Direct sowing in the ground or pots is recommended at a depth of about 1 cm. The plant is hardy and easy to care for, requiring regular but moderate watering. It flowers during summer and autumn, and its flowers can be harvested for use.

Parts used:
The parts of the marigold used are mainly the flowers. These are harvested when they are fully open and in full bloom. The flowers are dried and used in various forms, such as infusions, oils, ointments, or tinctures. They can also be used fresh in salads or other dishes.

Components:
It contains various beneficial components, including flavonoids, carotenoids, essential oils, phenolic acids, and triterpe-

nes, which give its medicinal and antioxidant properties.

History and tradition:
Calendula has a long history of use in folk medicine and herbal traditions. It has been prized for its medicinal properties and used to treat many conditions, including wounds, burns, skin inflammations, digestive problems and gynecological ailments. In addition, it has been considered a symbol of joy and prosperity in many cultures and is used in celebrations and rituals.

Therapeutic properties:
It is known for its therapeutic properties and health benefits. Some of the properties attributed to this plant include anti-inflammatory, healing, antiseptic, antioxidant, and soothing actions. It has been used topically to treat minor burns, cuts, abrasions, insect bites, eczema and dermatitis. Due to its moisturizing properties and ability to improve skin appearance, it has also been used in skin care products such as creams, lotions, and ointments.

Curiosities:
Calendula, commonly known as "marigold", is a medicinal plant renowned for its healing and cosmetic properties. Native to southern Europe, it is now cultivated in various regions worldwide. The bright orange flowers of calendula can be used fresh or dried to create infusions, oils, and creams.

Historically, it has been valued for its anti-inflammatory, healing, and antioxidant effects. It is frequently incorporated into cosmetics, such as creams, lotions, and other skincare products. Externally, calendula is used to treat various conditions, and as an infusion, it can help with digestive issues and regulate the menstrual cycle. Traditional medicine is also credited with antispasmodic, diuretic, and emmenagogue properties.

Adverse or side effects:
It is typically safe for topical use or as an infusion. However, some individuals may experience allergic reactions, such as redness, irritation, or skin itching. In rare cases, severe reactions can occur, including swelling of the face, lips, or tongue, difficulty breathing, or widespread skin rashes. If any of these symptoms arise, please seek medical attention immediately.

Contraindications:
It is generally considered safe for most people; however, there are some essential contraindications to remember. Individuals allergic to plants in the Asteraceae family—such as chrysanthemums, arnica, or daisies—may also be at a higher risk for allergic reactions to calendula and should avoid using it.

If you are pregnant or breastfeeding, consult a healthcare professional before using calendula products, as there is insufficient evidence regarding their safety during these periods. Additionally, if you have a scheduled surgery, it is best to avoid calendula, as it may affect blood clotting.

Interactions:
There have been no significant reported interactions between calendula and specific medications. However, it's always wise to consult a physician or pharmacist before combining calendula with other medicines. Since calendula may have anticoagulant properties, caution is essential when taking anticoagulant medications, such as warfarin, as this may increase the risk of bleeding. Additionally, if you are taking medicines for diabetes, be cautious, as calendula may lower blood sugar levels.

Chamomile (Matricaria chamomilla)

Description:
Chamomile is an annual herbaceous plant in the Asteraceae family. Its erect, branched stem can reach a height of up to 60 centimeters. The leaves are finely divided and light green. The flowers are small and daisy-shaped, with a yellow center surrounded by white petals. A distinctive apple scent is released when the flowers are rubbed between the fingers.

Habitat and cultivation:
Chamomile is native to Europe and commonly found in temperate climate regions. It grows best in well-drained, nutrient-rich soils and can be found in meadows, fields, roadsides and gardens. Chamomile is a hardy and adaptable plant that can grow in various conditions. It can also be quickly grown from seed or by dividing existing plants.

Parts used:
The dried flowers are used in the chamomile parts. These are harvested when fully open and air-dried to preserve their therapeutic properties. The dried flowers are used to prepare infusions, extracts, essential oils and cosmetic products.

Components:
Chamomile contains various components that contribute to its therapeutic properties. These include essential oils, such as bisabolol and azulene oxide, which have anti-inflammatory and soothing properties. It also contains flavonoids, such as apigenin, which have antioxidant and anti-inflammatory properties. Other components present in chamomile include caffeic acid, coumarins and polyphenols.

History and tradition:
Various cultures have used chamomile since ancient times due to its therapeutic properties. The ancient Egyptians used it in religious rituals and skin care. It was also known and used in traditional Greek and Roman medicine. In popular tradition, chamomile is associated with calming and relaxing properties and has been used to relieve stress, anxiety, and sleep disorders.

Therapeutic properties:
Chamomile is known for its therapeutic properties and is used in herbal medicine for its various health benefits. It is attributed to anti-inflammatory, antioxidant, antibacterial, soothing, and digestive properties. Chamomile is commonly used to relieve upset stomach, colic, indigestion and nausea. It is also used to relieve stress and anxiety and promote relaxation. In addition, it has been used topically to reduce skin irritation, minor burns, and skin conditions such as dermatitis and eczema.

Curiosities:
Chamomile (Matricaria chamomilla) is an herbaceous Asteraceae plant with exciting curiosities. For example, its name comes from the Greek "chamaimelon", which means "apple on earth", due to its characteristic apple aroma. In addition, chamomile has been used for centuries in multiple cultures for its therapeutic properties and is considered one of the oldest and most popular herbs in herbal medicine.

Adverse or side effects:
Chamomile is generally considered safe and well-tolerated. However, adverse effects or side effects may occur in some cases. Some people may experience allergic reactions when they contact the plant or consume chamomile products. In addition, excessive consumption may cause stomach upset, nausea, or vomiting. It is essential to be aware of these possible effects, discontinue use, and consult a health professional if you experience any.

Contraindications:
Although generally safe, it has some contraindications. For example, people who are allergic to other plants in the Asteraceae family, such as ragweed or sunflower, may be at increased risk of developing allergic reactions to chamomile. In addition, caution is advised in pregnant or nursing women, as not enough studies have been conducted to determine its safety in these stages.

Interactions:
In general, chamomile has not been associated with significant drug interactions. However, it is always advisable to consult a healthcare professional if you are taking any medications or have pre-existing health conditions before using chamomile therapeutically. Some studies suggest that chamomile may have mild anticoagulant effects, so caution should be exercised when combining it with anticoagulant or antiplatelet medications.

Fennel (Foeniculum vulgare)

Description:
Fennel is a perennial herbaceous plant in the Apiaceae family. Its erect, striated stems can reach a height of up to 2 meters. The leaves are long, finely divided, and bright green. The flowers are small, yellow, and grouped in umbels. Fennel produces dry, elongated fruits, which contain seeds. Both the leaves and seeds have a distinctive aroma and an anise flavor.

Habitat and cultivation:
Fennel is native to the Mediterranean region but is cultivated

in many parts of the world due to its culinary and medicinal value. It prefers well-drained, fertile soils and can grow in full sun or partial shade. It is drought-resistant and can tolerate cold temperatures. It quickly grows from seed and is found in gardens and commercial cultivation.

Parts used:
The parts of fennel used for culinary and medicinal purposes are the seeds, leaves, and stems. The seeds are the most commonly used, either whole or ground. The leaves and stems can also be fresh or dried to flavor dishes.

Components:
Fennel contains various beneficial health components. Its seeds are rich in essential oils, such as anethole, which give it its characteristic aroma and flavor. They also contain phenolic compounds, flavonoids and phytochemicals, which have antioxidant and anti-inflammatory properties. Fennel is also a good source of dietary fiber, vitamins (C and B6), and minerals (calcium, iron and potassium).

History and tradition:
Fennel has a long history of use in traditional medicine and cooking in different cultures. Indian Ayurvedic medicine treats digestive problems such as indigestion and colic. Traditional Chinese medicine improves digestion, relieves gas, and promotes breastfeeding. In addition, fennel has been used in Mediterranean cuisine since ancient times for its flavor and digestive properties.

Therapeutic properties:
Fennel has therapeutic properties that make it valuable in natural medicine. It has been used to relieve digestive problems, such as indigestion, colic, and flatulence. Due to its expectorant and antispasmodic properties, it has also been used to treat respiratory conditions, such as coughs and the common cold. Fennel has also been used to stimulate appetite, promote breastfeeding, and relieve symptoms of premenstrual syndrome. In addition, its potential to reduce inflammation, improve eye health, and promote cardiovascular health has been investigated. However, it is essential to note that fennel, such as

allergies, may adversely affect some people.

Curiosities:
Fennel has some interesting curiosities associated with its history and use. In ancient Greece, fennel was believed to be a sacred plant used in religious ceremonies. In addition, Greek and Roman warriors used to chew fennel seeds to increase their strength and endurance. In the Middle Ages, fennel was believed to have magical powers and was used as a talisman to protect against the evil eye and evil spells. In cooking, fennel is known for its use in traditional dishes such as fennel bread and liqueur, which are consumed in many Mediterranean countries.

Adverse or side effects:
Although fennel is generally considered safe for most people when consumed in moderate amounts, it may cause some adverse side effects in some individuals. Some people may experience allergies to fennel, which may manifest as skin rashes, itching, or difficulty breathing. In addition, excessive consumption of fennel may cause stomach upset, diarrhea, or a burning sensation in the stomach. In rare cases, severe allergic reactions have been reported, such as swelling of the face, lips, or tongue, requiring immediate medical attention.

Contraindications:
Although fennel is generally safe for most people, there are some contraindications. Pregnant women should avoid consuming it, as it may stimulate the uterus and cause contractions, which can be dangerous during pregnancy. Caution is also advised in lactating women, as it is unknown whether fennel consumption can affect breast milk produc-tion. People with blood clotting disorders or who are taking anticoagulants should avoid fennel, as it may increase the risk of bleeding.

Interactions:
Fennel may interact with some medications, so it is essential to use caution when combining it with other treatments. For example, fennel may increase the effects of anticoagulant drugs, such as warfarin, increasing the risk of bleeding. In addition, fennel may interfere with the absorption of certain medications,

such as proton pump inhibitors used to treat heartburn or thyroid medications. It has also been reported that it may have a weak estrogenic effect, so people who take hormone therapy or have a history of hormone-related cancer should use caution and consult their physician before using fennel.

Ginger (Zingiber officinale)

Description:
It is a perennial plant with underground stems called rhizomes. It has long, narrow leaves and yellow or white cone-shaped flowers. The rhizome is the most commonly used part and has a spicy and aromatic flavor.

Habitat and cultivation:
Ginger is native to tropical Asia and is grown in many parts of the world. It prefers warm, humid climates and can be grown both in gardens and in pots indoors.

Parts used:
The rhizome of ginger is the most commonly used part. It is harvested, peeled, and used fresh or dried for culinary and medicinal purposes. The leaves and flowers can also be used in specific preparations.

Components:
Ginger contains active compounds such as gingerol, shogaol and zingiberene, which give it medicinal properties. It also contains antioxidants, vitamins and minerals.

Ginger is a perennial plant native to tropical Asia. Due to its multiple health benefits, it has been used for centuries as a spice in cooking and traditional medicine.

History and tradition:
This plant has been cultivated and used in Asia for over 5,000 years. It is believed to have originated in the coastal region of South Asia, specifically in what we today know as India and China. From there, it spread to various parts of the world and was integrated into many cultures' culinary and medicinal

traditions.

Ginger is especially valued in traditional Asian medicine, such as Ayurvedic and Chinese medicine. In these traditions, it is considered a "hot" plant that can help balance the body and treat various ailments. It has been used to relieve digestive problems, such as nausea, vomiting and upset stomach. In addition, it has been used as a general tonic to strengthen the immune system and promote blood circulation.

Therapeutic properties:

Ginger contains bioactive compounds, such as gingerols and shogaols, which give it medicinal properties. These com- pounds are responsible for ginger's characteristic flavor and aroma and benefit the human body.

One of ginger's best-known properties is its ability to relieve nausea and vomiting. Numerous studies have shown that ginger consumption can effectively relieve nausea caused by surgery, pregnancy, or chemotherapy. The compounds in ginger act on the digestive system, reducing discomfort and improving intestinal motility.

In addition, ginger has also been used to relieve pain and inflammation. Gingerols and shogaols have been shown to have anti-inflammatory and analgesic properties, making them a natural choice for pain relief in conditions such as arthritis, muscle aches and migraines. Some studies even suggest that regular consumption of ginger may help reduce chronic inflammation in the body.

Ginger may also have positive effects on cardiovascular health. It has been suggested that regular consumption of ginger may help reduce cholesterol and triglyceride levels in the blood and improve blood circulation. These effects could contribute to heart health and reduce the risk of cardio-vascular disease.

Curiosities:

Ginger, whose scientific name is Zingiber officinale, is a plant native to tropical Asia. It has been used for centuries in cooking and traditional medicine due to its medicinal properties. Here are some interesting facts about ginger:

Spicy and refreshing flavor: Ginger has a distinctive taste with a spicy and refreshing touch. This characteristic flavor is due to active compounds such as gingerols and shogaols, which also give it its medicinal properties.

Ancient use: Ginger has been used in traditional Chinese and Indian medicine for over 2,000 years to treat various conditions, from digestive problems to muscle aches and colds.

Culinary use: It is a popular cooking spice. Besides its medicinal properties, it is used in sweet and savory dishes, such as curries, desserts, infusions, and refreshing drinks like ginger ale.

Adverse or side effects:

Although ginger is generally safe for most people when consumed in moderate amounts, some people may experience adverse side effects:

Upset stomach: Excessive consumption of ginger may cause an upset stomach, nausea, heartburn, or diarrhea in some people. These side effects are usually mild and go away on their own.

Interference with medications: Ginger may interact with certain medications, such as anticoagulants or antihypertensives. Caution is advised when combining ginger with these medications; it is crucial to consult a physician.

Allergic reactions: Although rare, some people may be allergic to ginger. These reactions may manifest as skin rashes, itching, swelling, or difficulty breathing. If you experience any allergic reactions, seek medical attention immediately.

Contraindications:

There are contraindications to take into account when using it:

Coagulation disorders: Because ginger inhibits platelet aggregation, caution should be exercised in people with coagulation disorders or who take anticoagulant drugs. A physician should be consulted before use.

Pregnancy and lactation: Although it has traditionally been used to treat nausea during pregnancy, caution is advised during these stages. A physician should be consulted before use.

Interactions:

It can interact with certain medications and supplements, so it is essential to use caution when combining it with other treatments. Some known interactions include:

Anticoagulants: Ginger, which inhibits platelet aggregation, may increase the risk of bleeding when combined with anticoagulant medications such as warfarin. Medical supervision is recommended if both treatments are used.

Antihypertensives: Ginger may have hypotensive effects, which could interact with high blood pressure medications. If you are taking medicines for hypertension, exercise caution and consult a physician before using ginger.

Green anise (Pimpinella anisum)

Description:
Green anise is an annual herbaceous plant in the Apiaceae family. It is native to the Mediterranean region and has spread to other parts of the world due to its popularity as a spice and medicinal plant. The plant has green, feathery leaves and produces small, white, umbel-shaped flowers. Its small and oval-shaped fruits contain seeds used for culinary and medicinal purposes. The plant has a sweet and distinctive aroma.

Habitat and cultivation:
Green anise grows best in warm, sunny climates. It prefers well-drained and fertile soils. It is grown in many parts of the world, including the Mediterranean, Europe, Asia and North America. Green anise can be grown from seed and requires proper care to ensure healthy growth.

Parts used:
The parts used of green anise are the ripe seeds, which are harvested when the fruits are fully ripe. The seeds are dried and used whole or ground in culinary and medicinal preparations.

Components:
It contains various chemical compounds that give it therapeutic properties and a distinctive flavor. Some main components include essential oils (such as anethole), flavonoids, coumarins and phenolic compounds. These compounds are responsible for green anise's characteristic aroma, flavor, and medicinal properties.

History and tradition:
Green anise has been used in various cultures since ancient

times. The Egyptians reportedly used it in religious rituals, while the Romans and Greeks used it as a spice and remedy for digestive problems. In traditional medicine, green anise has been used to treat digestive disorders, colic, and respiratory issues, as well as an appetite stimulant.

Therapeutic properties:
Green anise has several therapeutic properties, making it valuable in traditional medicine and aromatherapy. Some of its key benefits include:
- Relieving gas and abdominal bloating
- Stimulating the production of digestive enzymes and promoting proper digestion
- Alleviating chest congestion and facilitating expectoration
- Soothing muscle spasms and easing colic
- Stimulating breast milk production in lactating women

Additionally, the compounds in green anise possess antimicrobial and antioxidant properties, which help combat infections and protect against oxidative damage.

Curiosities:
Green anise has been used as a medicinal plant and spice for thousands of years. Ancient Egyptians reportedly used it to treat digestive ailments and in religious rituals. Green anise is commonly used in cooking to flavor various dishes and baked goods. It also manufactures alcoholic beverages, such as ouzo, raki and absinthe. In some cultures, green anise symbolizes good luck and is believed to have aphrodisiac properties.

Adverse or side effects:
Green anise is generally safe to consume in moderate amounts. However, some individuals may experience adverse effects, such as allergic reactions, gastrointestinal irritation, skin rashes, or difficulty breathing. In rare cases, green anise can cause increased sensitivity to sunlight, raising the risk of sunburn. If consumed in large quantities, it is advisable to use sunscreen and limit sun exposure. Additionally, excessive consumption may lead to a laxative effect and result in diarrhea.

Contraindications:
Individuals allergic to anise or plants from the Apiaceae family

(such as fennel, celery, or dill) should avoid consuming green anise, as they may experience allergic reactions. Additionally, green anise may act as a uterine stimulant, so pregnant women should avoid it, as it could increase the risk of uterine contractions. Those with gastric ulcers, inflam-matory bowel disease, or bleeding disorders should also limit their intake of green anise, as it may exacerbate these conditions.

Interactions:
Green anise may interact with certain medications, including anticoagulants and antiplatelet agents, which can increase the risk of bleeding. It is advisable to consult a physician if you are taking these drugs. Additionally, green anise may have a mild sedative effect, potentially enhancing the effects of sedative or anesthetic medications. Therefore, caution is recommended if you are taking such medications. Furthermore, green anise may interfere with the metabolism of drugs processed by the liver, such as certain cholesterol-lowering medications and oral contraceptives, which could decrease their effectiveness.

Lemon balm (Melissa officinalis)

Description:
Lemon balm is a perennial herbaceous plant in the Lamiaceae family. Its quadrangular, branched stem can reach a height of up to 70 centimeters. The leaves are opposite, oval, toothed, and light green. The small, white or pink flowers are grouped in terminal spikes. Rubbing the leaves between the fingers gives off a fresh citrus scent.

Habitat and cultivation:
Lemon balm is native to the Mediterranean region, although it is now cultivated in various parts of the world. It grows best in well-drained, nutrient-rich soils. It can be found in gardens, roadsides, and wild areas. Lemon balm is a hardy and adaptable plant that can grow in various conditions. It is easily propagated through seed, cuttings, or division of existing plants.

Parts used:
The parts of lemon balm used are the leaves and stems. These

are harvested when the plant is in full bloom and are air-dried to preserve their therapeutic properties. The dried leaves and stems are used to prepare infusions, tinctures, essential oils and cosmetic products.

Components:
Lemon balm contains various components that give it its therapeutic properties. These include essential oils, such as citronellal, citral and geraniol, which give it its characteristic citrus aroma and have sedative and calming properties. It also contains flavonoids, such as luteolin and apigenin, which have antioxidant and anti-inflammatory properties. Other components present in lemon balm include rosmarinic acid, polyphenols and tannins.

History and tradition:
Various cultures have used Lemon balm since ancient times due to its therapeutic properties. In ancient Greece, properties were attributed to relieving stress and anxiety and promoting relaxation. It was also known as the "elixir of youth" due to its ability to calm the heart and improve mood. In traditional European medicine, lemon balm has been used to treat sleep disorders, digestive problems and nervous system conditions.

Therapeutic properties:
Lemon balm is known for its therapeutic properties and is used in herbal medicine for its various health benefits. It is attributed with sedative, calming, antispasmodic, carminative, and digestive properties. Lemon balm is commonly used to relieve stress, anxiety, and insomnia and promote relaxation. It also reduces digestive disorders such as indigestion, gas and colic. In addition, it has been used topically to relieve skin irritation, insect bites and mild skin conditions.

Curiosities:
Melissa has been used since ancient times for its therapeutic properties, but it also has some exciting curiosities. For example, its scientific name, Melissa officinalis, comes from the Greek "melissa", which means bee. This plant attracts bees due to its aroma and nectar. Another curious fact is that lemon balm has been traditionally used as an insect repellent, especially

against mosquitoes and flies. In addition, due to its pleasant citrus aroma, it has been used to manufacture perfumes and cosmetic products.

Adverse or side effects:
Lemon balm is generally considered safe when used correctly and in appropriate doses. However, some people may experience adverse effects. These may include gastrointestinal irritation, such as nausea, vomiting, or diarrhea, especially when consumed in large amounts. Skin allergies have also been reported in people sensitive to the plant. In sporadic cases, excessive sedative effects or drowsiness have been reported in some people. If any of these adverse effects are experienced, it is advisable to discontinue using lemon balm and consult a health professional.

Contraindications:
Although lemon balm is generally considered safe, there are some contraindications. Its use is not recommended in pregnant or breastfeeding women, as there is not enough evidence about its safety in these cases. People who are allergic to other plants of the Lamiaceae family, such as mint or oregano, should also exercise caution, as they may be more prone to developing allergic reactions. In addition, due to its sedative properties, it is recommended to avoid its consumption before driving or performing activities that require attention and concentration.

Interactions:
Lemon balm may interact with certain medications and herbs, so caution is advised when taking other treatments. It may enhance the sedative effects of sleeping medications or tranquilizers, causing excessive drowsiness. It may also interact with anticoagulant drugs, such as warfarin, increasing the risk of bleeding. Therefore, it is advisable to consult your doctor before combining lemon balm with other medications or herbs to avoid possible interactions.

Licorice or Liquorice (Glycyrrhiza glabra)

Description:

Licorice, scientifically known as Glycyrrhiza glabra, is a perennial plant that belongs to the legume family. It has an erect and branched stem, which can reach a height of up to 1 meter. Its leaves are pinnate, with elongated leaflets, and are bright green. The flowers of licorice are small and violet or pale blue, grouped in clusters. The most used part of the plant is its root, which is thick, fibrous, and dark brown.

Habitat and cultivation:
Licorice is native to warm, temperate regions of Europe and Asia but is now cultivated in various parts of the world. It prefers well-drained, fertile soils and can grow in sunny and semi-shaded areas. The plant requires a climate with moderate temperatures and a good amount of water for optimal growth. Licorice can be propagated by seed or by root division.

Parts used:
The most commonly used part of the licorice plant is its root, which contains most of its beneficial components. However, the leaves and stems can also be used to a lesser extent, although they are rare. The root is harvested when the plant is at least three years old, usually in autumn, and dried for later use.

Components:
Licorice root contains a variety of health-promoting components. One of the main components is glycyrrhizin, a compound that gives it its characteristic sweet taste. It also contains flavonoids, saponins, coumarins, essential oils and phytosterols. These compounds have antioxidant, anti-inflammatory, antimicrobial, and antiviral properties.

History and tradition:
Licorice has a long history of use in traditional medicine in various cultures. It is believed to have been first used in ancient Mesopotamia more than 4,000 years ago. The Egyptians, Greeks and Romans all valued licorice for its medicinal properties and sweet taste. In traditional Chinese medicine, licorice has been used for centuries as a tonic for the respiratory and digestive systems. Due to its sweet and characteristic flavor, licorice has also been used to manufacture candies, sweets and confectionery products.

Therapeutic properties:
Licorice has many therapeutic properties that make it valuable in natural medicine. It is mainly used as an anti-inflammatory, expectorant, and digestive. Due to its expectorant and lung-soothing properties, it has been used to relieve respiratory conditions, such as colds, coughs, bronchitis and asthma. It also reduces digestive problems like heartburn, indigestion, ulcers, and spasms. In addition, licorice has traditionally been used as a tonic for the liver, kidneys, and adrenal glands. However, it is essential to note that, due to its glycyrrhizin content, excessive and prolonged consumption of licorice may have adverse effects, especially in people with certain health conditions, such as hypertension or kidney failure. Therefore, it is advisable to use licorice with caution and under the supervision of a health professional.

Curiosities:
Licorice, or Glycyrrhiza glabra, is a perennial plant used for various historical purposes. An interesting fact about licorice is its scientific name, which comes from Greek and means "sweet root". This is because licorice root has a sweet taste and has traditionally been used as a natural sweetener in various culinary preparations and medicinal products. In addition, licorice has also been used to manufacture tobacco products, such as cigarettes and chewing gum.

Adverse or side effects:
Although licorice is considered safe when consumed in moderate amounts, excessive consumption may have adverse effects. One of the main components of licorice is glycyrrhizin, which can cause fluid retention and raise blood pressure in some people. This can be especially worrisome for those who already suffer from hypertension or heart problems. In addition, prolonged and excessive consumption of licorice can cause electrolyte imbalances, such as decreased potassium levels in the body. Cases of kidney and hormone damage have also been reported in people who have consumed large amounts of licorice over prolonged periods.

Contraindications:
Licorice has some crucial contraindications that need to be

taken into account. Its consumption is not recommended for pregnant women since glycyrrhizin can cross the placenta and affect the fetus. It is also not recommended during breast-feeding, as some components can pass into breast milk. In addition, people suffering from hypertension, heart disease, kidney failure, hormonal disorders, or diabetes should avoid or limit consumption of licorice due to possible adverse effects.

Interactions:
It may interact with certain medications and herbs, enhancing or diminishing their effect. For example, consumption of licorice may increase the effects of medicines used to treat hypertension, which can lead to a dangerous drop in blood pressure. It may also interact with blood-thinning medications, such as warfarin, and increase the risk of bleeding. In addition, licorice may interfere with some medicines used to treat diabetes, as it can affect blood sugar levels. Therefore, it is essential to consult a healthcare professional before combining licorice with other medications or herbs to avoid possible interactions.

Mallow (Malva sylvestris)

Description:
Mallow is a perennial herbaceous plant in the Malvaceae family. Its erect, branched stem can reach a height of up to 1 meter. Its leaves are large, palmate and toothed, bright green. The funnel-shaped flowers vary in color from pale pink to deep purple. This plant is known for its beauty and is used in ornamental gardens and traditional medicine.

Habitat and cultivation:
Mallow is native to Europe and is commonly found in meadows, roadsides and wastelands. It adapts to different types of soils, although it prefers well-drained, nutrient-rich soils. This plant can grow in temperate and warm climates, tolerating direct sun and partial shade. Mallow is easily propagated by seed and can also be grown from cuttings.

Parts used:
Mallow leaves and flowers are mainly used for medicinal

purposes. The leaves are harvested when the plant is fully grown, while the flowers are harvested when fully open. The dried parts of the plant are then used to prepare infusions, extracts, or ointments.

Components:
Mallow contains several bioactive components that give it its therapeutic properties. Among them are mucilages, gel-like substances with emollient and softening properties. It also contains flavonoids, antioxidants, and phenolic compounds, which have anti-inflammatory and antioxidant effects.

History and tradition:
Mallow has been used in traditional medicine for centuries. Ancient Egyptians and Greeks, for example, are believed to have used it to treat various conditions, such as respiratory diseases, skin irritations and digestive problems. In addition, in some traditions, it is considered a sacred plant attributed to its protective and magical properties.

Therapeutic properties:
Mallow is used in herbal medicine because of its therapeutic properties. It is attributed with anti-inflammatory, emollient, soothing, and healing properties. Therefore, it treats respiratory conditions such as coughs and colds and digestive problems such as gastritis and heartburn. It is also used topically to relieve skin irritation such as minor burns, rashes and insect bites.

Curiosities:
Mallow, also known as Malva sylvestris, is an herbaceous perennial plant with some exciting characteristics. It has been used since ancient times for its medicinal properties and was attributed with magical and protective properties. In addition, this plant is known for its beauty, as it produces showy flowers in shades ranging from light pink to deep purple.

Adverse or side effects:
Although mallow is generally considered safe, adverse or side effects may occur in rare cases. Some people may experience allergic reactions when coming into contact with the plant or consuming its parts. In addition, excessive consumption of

mallow may have a laxative effect and cause diarrhea. It is important to note that, as with any medicinal plant, it is advisable to use it in moderation and consult a health professional if adverse effects occur.

Contraindications:
Mallow has no significant contraindications, but caution is advised in some instances. For example, people with a history of allergies or sensitivity to other plants of the Malvaceae family may be at increased risk of allergic reactions to mallow. In addition, it is advised to avoid using mallow during pregnancy and breastfeeding, as not enough studies have been conducted to determine its safety in these stages.

Interactions:
Mallow has not been associated with significant drug or supplement interactions. However, it is always advisable to consult a healthcare professional if you are taking any medications or have pre-existing health conditions before using Mallow therapeutically. This is especially relevant if you take anticoagulants or other drugs that may interact with herbs or medicinal plants.

Marshmallow (Althaea officinalis)

Description:
Marshmallow (Althaea officinalis) is a perennial herbaceous plant in the Malvaceae family. Its erect, hairy stem can reach a height of up to 1.5 meters. The leaves are large, lobed, and toothed, and dark green. The marshmallow flowers are large and showy, with five petals in shades ranging from white to light pink or purple. The plant has a thick, fleshy taproot used for medicinal purposes.

Habitat and cultivation:
Marshmallow is native to Europe and grows in moist areas such as riverbanks and ponds. It prefers nutrient-rich, well-drained soils and is cold-hardy but can grow in warmer climates. Marshmallows can be propagated through seed or root division. This hardy plant can quickly grow in gardens and orchards.

Parts used:
The marshmallow root is the most commonly used medicinal ingredient. It is harvested in autumn when the plant has completed its growth cycle and the leaves have fallen. The root is dried and used to prepare infusions, extracts and ointments. The leaves and flowers can also be used, although to a lesser extent.

Components:
It contains several active components that give it its medicinal properties. Among them are mucilages and gelatinous substances that are emollient and softening. It also contains flavonoids, tannins, phenolic acids, and allantoin, which have anti-inflammatory, antioxidant, and healing properties.

History and tradition:
Since ancient times, marshmallows have been used for medicinal and culinary purposes. The Egyptians and Greeks used it to treat respiratory, digestive, and skin conditions. In addition, in popular tradition, marshmallows are believed to have protective properties and ward off evil spirits. They are also attributed to aphrodisiac properties and have been used in love and fertility rituals.

Therapeutic properties:
This plant is used in herbal medicine due to its therapeutic properties. It is attributed with anti-inflammatory, emollient, soothing, and healing properties. Therefore, it relieves irritation and inflammation of the throat, cough, cold, bronchitis, and digestive problems such as gastritis and ulcers. It is also topically used to reduce skin irritation, minor burns, insect bites, and wounds.

Curiosities:
Marshmallow, also known as Althaea officinalis, has some exciting curiosities. For example, its scientific name, Althaea, is derived from the Greek word "cure" or "healing", reflecting its long history of medicinal use. In addition, marshmallows have traditionally been used to make soft, sticky candies from the plant's root. These candies were named after the marshmallow because of their smooth, sticky texture.

Adverse or side effects:
Although it is generally considered safe, adverse or side effects may occur in rare cases. Some people may experience allergic reactions when coming into contact with the plant or consuming its parts. In addition, excessive marshmallow consumption may have a laxative effect and cause diarrhea. It is important to note that, as with any medicinal plant, it is advisable to use it in moderation and consult a health professional if adverse effects occur.

Contraindications:
There are no significant contraindications, but caution is advised in some instances. For example, people with a history of allergies or sensitivity to other plants in the Malvaceae family may be at increased risk of allergic reactions to marshmallows. In addition, marshmallows should not be used during pregnancy and breastfeeding, as not enough studies have been conducted to determine their safety in these stages.

Interactions:
Marshmallows have not been associated with significant drug or supplement interactions. However, it is always advisable to consult a healthcare professional if you take any medications or have pre-existing health conditions before using marshmallows therapeutically. This is especially relevant if you are taking anticoagulants or other drugs that may interact with herbs or medicinal plants.

Rosemary (Rosmarinus officinalis)

Description:
Rosemary is a perennial plant of the Lamiaceae family. It has small, linear, dark green leaves covered with a fine layer of hairs. It can reach a height of up to 1 meter and is characterized by its distinctive aroma and pleasantly bitter taste.

Habitat and cultivation:
It is native to the Mediterranean region but has spread to other parts of the world due to its popularity as an ornamental and culinary plant. It grows in well-drained, sunny soils and tolerates

dry and hot conditions. It can be grown from seed, cuttings, or bush division. It is a hardy and easy-to-maintain plant.

Parts used:
Both rosemary leaves and flowers are widely used. The leaves are harvested before flowering to obtain the maximum concentration of beneficial compounds, while the flowers are also harvested and used to a lesser extent.

Constituents:
It contains various beneficial chemical constituents, including essential oils (such as cineol, camphor and pinene), flavonoids, phenolic acids, and antioxidants, contributing to its therapeutic properties.

History and tradition:
Rosemary has a long history of use in cooking and traditional medicine. It has been appreciated since ancient times for its aromatic properties and has been attributed to symbolic and mystical qualities. In many cultures, it has been used in rituals and ceremonies to purify and protect.

Therapeutic properties:
Rosmary has several therapeutic properties. It has been traditionally used as a tonic for the nervous system, helping to improve memory and concentration. It is also attributed to digestive, stimulant, and antioxidant properties. It has been used externally to relieve muscle and joint pain and promote blood circulation.

Curiosities:
Rosemary has traditionally been considered a symbol of love and fidelity. In some cultures, it has been used in wedding ceremonies as a sign of good luck and protection. In ancient Greece, it was believed to strengthen memory and was associated with the goddess of love and beauty, Aphrodite. During the Middle Ages, it was thought to have protective powers against the evil eye, spirits, and disease.

Adverse or side effects:
In general, moderate dietary intake is safe for most people.

However, excessive doses may cause gastrointestinal irritation, headache, or dizziness. Some sensitive people may experience skin irritation from rosemary oil applied topically. Before using it extensively, it is recommended that a small amount be tested on a small area. Rosemary essential oil should not be ingested without medical supervision, as it can be toxic in high doses.

Contraindications:
It is not recommended for pregnant women, as it may stimulate uterine contractions and potentially induce premature labor. People suffering from epilepsy or seizures should avoid excessive consumption, as certain compounds may trigger episodes in sensitive individuals. Those with a known allergy to plants in the Lamiaceae family, such as mint, sage, or basil, may be more likely to react to rosemary.

Interactions:
It may interact with certain drugs, such as anticoagulants (e.g., warfarin) or antiplatelet drugs, increasing the risk of bleeding. Caution and medical consultation are recommended if taking any of these drugs. Due to its stimulant properties, rosemary may interfere with sedative or sleep-inducing medications, decreasing their effectiveness. If you take blood pressure medication, rosemary may have an additional effect on lowering blood pressure, which should be carefully monitored.

Yarrow (Achillea millefolium)

Description:
Yarrow is a perennial herbaceous plant belonging to the Asteraceae family. It is characterized by finely divided leaves and small flowers grouped in white, pink, or yellow corymbs. It reaches an average height of 30 to 60 centimeters and is widely distributed in temperate regions of Europe, Asia and North America.

Habitat and cultivation:
Yarrow is adaptable to various habitats, including meadows, hillsides, fields, roadsides and gardens. It prefers well-drained,

sunny soils but can also grow in partial shade. It is a hardy plant that can tolerate adverse conditions like drought and cold.

For cultivation, yarrow can be propagated by seed or bush division. Seeds are sown in spring or autumn, and young plants are transplanted once they reach a suitable size. The plant requires regular watering during its first year of growth, but thereafter, it is pretty hardy and does not need intensive maintenance.

Parts used:
Various parts of the yarrow are used for medicinal and cosmetic purposes. The most commonly used parts are the flowers and leaves harvested during the flowering season. The plant can be dried as infusions, tinctures, essential oils, or extracts.

Components:
It contains various chemical constituents that give it its medicinal properties. Among the most prominent are essential oils, such as azulene, borneol, cineol and chamazulene. It also contains flavonoids, sesquiterpenes, lactones, tannins and alkaloids.

History and tradition:
Yarrow has a long history of use in traditional medicine. It has been used in Europe and Asia as a medicinal plant for centuries to treat various conditions, such as digestive disorders, wounds, fever, menstrual cramps and respiratory problems. In addition, in some cultures, it has been associated with mystical properties and used in rituals and amulets for protection.

Therapeutic properties:
It has been valued for its therapeutic properties. Some properties attributed to this plant include anti-inflammatory, antispasmodic, diuretic, emmenagogue (menstrual flow stimulant), cicatrizant, and vulnerary (aid in wound healing) actions. It has also been used to relieve headaches, digestive disorders, fever and circulatory problems.

Curiosities:
The scientific name of yarrow, *Achillea millefolium*, is derived from the Greek hero Achilles. According to legend,

Achilles used yarrow to treat the wounds of his soldiers during the Trojan War. Due to its bitter taste and aromatic properties, yarrow has been used in producing beer and liquors, such as vermouth. It is an attractive plant for butterflies and other pollinators, making it a popular choice for wildlife and flower gardens. Historically, yarrow has also been used to repel insects like fleas and mosquitoes. Its leaves have been placed in closets and beds to help ward off these pests.

Adverse or side effects:
When used correctly, yarrow is generally considered safe. However, some people, especially those with sensitive skin, may experience mild side effects like skin irritation. Rarely, allergic reactions, such as skin rashes or difficulty breathing, have been reported in people sensitive to Asteraceae family plants. Caution is advised in pregnant or breastfeeding and young children since there is insufficient evidence of its safety in these groups.

Contraindications:
People with known allergies to Asteraceae family plants, such as daisies, or chrysanthemums, should avoid using yarrow, as they may have allergic reactions. Yarrow may have emmenagogue properties, which can stimulate menstrual flow. Therefore, pregnant women should avoid using it, as it may interfere with pregnancy. Caution is also advised in people taking anticoagulant medications or who have coagulation disorders, as yarrow may have a mild anticoagulant effect.

Interactions:
Yarrow may interact with some medications and herbs. It may increase the risk of bleeding when combined with anticoagulants or antiplatelet drugs, such as warfarin or aspirin. It has also been reported that yarrow may interact with sedative or hypnotic drugs, increasing the sedative effects. Caution is advised when combining it with these medications. If you are taking any medications or have a medical condition, it is essential to consult with a healthcare professional before starting Yarrow to avoid unwanted interactions.

BIBLIOGRAPHY & SCIENTIFIC STUDIES

1. "Plantas medicinales: El Dioscórides renovado" - Pío Font Quer
2. "Herbal Medicine: Biomolecular and Clinical Aspects" - Iris F. F. Benzie y Sissi Wachtel-Galor
3. "The Essential Guide to Herbal Safety" - Simon Y. Mills and Kerry Bone
4. "Guía de remedios naturales" - Andrew Chevallier
5. "Phytotherapy: A Quick Reference to Herbal Medicine" - Francesco Capasso, Luigi M. G. Gaginella, Angelo A. Izzo, y Naoki Mascolo
6. "Principles and Practice of Phytotherapy: Modern Herbal Medicine" - Simon Mills and Kerry Bone
7. "Herbal Medicine, Healing & Cancer" - Donald Yance
8. "Tratado de fitoterapia" - Juan Carlos Martín Montañez
9. "El gran libro de los remedios naturales" - Óscar López
10. "The Complete Herbal Tutor: The Definitive Guide to the Principles and Practices of Herbal Medicine" - Anne McIntyre
11. "Plantas medicinales y aromáticas: Cultivo, transformación y aplicaciones" - Javier Vallejo Ron
12. "The Encyclopedia of Medicinal Plants" - Andrew Chevallier
13. "The New Healing Herbs: The Classic Guide to Nature's Best Medicines" - Michael Castleman
14. "Fitoterapia: Vademécum de Prescripción" - Antonio López González
15. "Medicinal Plants: Chemistry and Properties" - David S. Seigler
16. "Remedios caseros con hierbas medicinales" - María Tránsito López
17. "Natural Remedies Encyclopedia" - Vance Ferrell
18. "A Modern Herbal" - Maud Grieve
19. "El poder curativo de las plantas" - Anne Iburg
20. "Herbal Antivirals: Natural Remedies for Emerging & Resistant Viral Infections" - Stephen Harrod Buhner

SCIENTIFIC STUDIES
1. "Curcumin: A Review of Its' Effects on Human Health" - Susan J. Hewlings and Douglas S. Kalman
2. "Curcumin, an atoxic antioxidant and natural NFκB, cyclooxygenase-2, lipooxygenase, and inducible nitric oxide synthase inhibitor: A shield against acute and chronic diseases" - Bharat B. Aggarwal, Harikumar KB
3. "Curcumin for Inflammatory Bowel Disease: A Review of Human Studies" - K. Lang, D. L. Denson
4. "Glutamine and the Regulation of Intestinal Permeability: From Bench to Bedside" - Josef Neu, Doug M. Mshar
5. "Glutamine Supplementation in Gastrointestinal Diseases" - M. Papaléo, A. M. Faintuch
6. "The role of glutamine in protecting against gastric mucosal

damage: An experimental study" - Hiroshi Okabe, Hiromi Hashimoto
7. "Ginger in gastrointestinal disorders: A systematic review of clinical trials" - R. Haniadka, Z. A. Rajeev
8. "Ginger: An Overview of Health Benefits" - Ann Bode, Zigang Dong
9. "Ginger and Its Constituents: Role in Prevention and Treatment of Gastrointestinal Cancer" - R. Sharma, S. K. Gescher
10. "Chamomile: A herbal medicine of the past with bright future" - Srivastava JK, Shankar E, Gupta S
11. "The effect of chamomile extract on the prevention of Helicobacter pylori infection" - A. Mahady, G. Pendland
12. "Chamomile: An ancient pain remedy and a modern gout medication" - M. McKay, J. Blumberg
13. "The Role of Probiotics in the Treatment of Helicobacter pylori Infection" - D. L. Mack, G. D. Reid
14. "Probiotics for Gastrointestinal Conditions: A Summary of the Evidence" - J. B. Ritchie, M. G. Romanuk
15. "Probiotics in the Management of Gastritis: A Review" - S. B. Goldin, H. S. Gorbach
16. "Licorice Extracts in the Treatment of Functional Dyspepsia and Gastritis" - A. H. Kang, S. L. Lee
17. "The Effects of Licorice Extract on Gastric Mucosal Protection in Rats" - M. Armanini, A. Fiore
18. "Glycyrrhizin and Its Metabolites: Potential Sources of Naturally Occurring Antiviral Agents" - H. Pompei, L. R. Floreani
19. "Vitamin B12 and Gastritis: A Review of the Evidence" - J. L. Allen, C. M. L. Stabler
20. "Vitamin B12 as a Treatment for Gastritis: Case Studies and Clinical Trials" - H. N. Herbert, R. W. Snow
21. "The Role of Vitamin B12 in Gastric Mucosal Health" - M. Lindenbaum, J. M. Healton
22. "Zinc and Gastrointestinal Health: Current Evidence for Zinc Supplementation in Gastritis" - S. Prasad, J. Beck
23. "Zinc in the Management of Gastric Ulcers: A Review" - M. J. Hambidge, N. F. Krebs
24. "Zinc: An Essential Micronutrient for Gastrointestinal Health" - L. Gibson, J. Ferguson
25. "Aloe Vera in the Management of Gastritis: A Review of the Evidence" - T. Reynolds, A. C. Dweck
26. "The Therapeutic Potential of Aloe Vera in the Treatment of Gastric Ulcers" - B. B. Singh, M. S. Levine
27. "Aloe Vera and Its Therapeutic Efficacy in Treating Gastric Mucosal Disorders" - J. Grindlay, T. Reynolds
28. "Aniseed and Its Role in Gastrointestinal Health: A Review" - C. L. Bisset, H. Wichtl
29. "The Efficacy of Aniseed in the Treatment of Functional Dyspepsia" - R. M. C. Hill, D. L. Newmark
30. "Anise Oil and Its Beneficial Effects on the Gastrointestinal System" - A. L. Miller, J. P. Smith
31. "Boldo in the Treatment of Gastrointestinal Disorders: A Review" - J. A. Duke, M. J. Bogenschutz-Godwin
32. "Pharmacological Properties of Boldo: Emphasis on Digestive Benefits" - L. R. Cechinel-Filho, H. A. Yunes

33. "The Role of Boldo in the Management of Digestive Health" - P. G. Waterman, S. Mole
34. "Calendula as a Herbal Remedy for Gastritis: A Comprehensive Review" - E. Della Loggia, S. Tubaro
35. "Antioxidant and Anti-inflammatory Properties of Calendula for Gastric Health" - M. Preethi, N. Kuttan
36. "Calendula and Its Efficacy in Treating Gastric Ulcers" - R. García, J. C. Carrasco
37. "Fennel and Its Gastrointestinal Benefits: A Review" - A. Badgujar, V. Jain
38. "The Role of Fennel in Managing Gastrointestinal Disorders" - S. E. McKay, J. M. Blumberg
39. "Fennel as a Herbal Treatment for Gastritis: Evidence and Mechanisms" - A. N. Dhiman, V. R. Sharma
40. "Anti-inflammatory and Gastroprotective Effects of Mallow on Gastric Mucosa" - F. Conforti, S. Sosa
41. "Mallow Extracts in the Management of Gastritis: A Review" - L. Barros, P. Baptista
42. "The Role of Mallow in Gastric Health: Evidences from Clinical Studies" - M. S. M. Júnior, A. M. L. Silva
43. "The Use of Marshmallow Root in the Treatment of Gastritis: A Review" - C. A. Newall, L. A. Anderson
44. "Marshmallow Root and Its Gastroprotective Properties" - R. J. Houghton, A. Zarka
45. "Effects of Marshmallow Root Extract on Gastric Mucosal Protection" - T. P. Brown, J. D. Dattner
46. "Melissa and Its Role in Gastrointestinal Health: An Overview" - M. Kennedy, N. Scholey
47. "The Efficacy of Lemon Balm in the Treatment of Gastric Disorders" - S. C. Awad, J. A. Levick
48. "Melissa Officinalis: Potential Benefits for Gastric Health" - E. A. Perry, M. S. Bollen
49. "Yarrow and Its Gastroprotective Properties: A Review" - K. S. C. Kumar, R. Bhowmik
50. "The Use of Yarrow in the Treatment of Gastric Ulcers" - L. K. Ghazanfari, M. A. Minae
51. "Yarrow Extracts: Potential Applications in Gastritis Management" - J. M. Vázquez, R. A. Morales
52. "Rosemary and Its Gastrointestinal Benefits: A Comprehensive Review" - R. A. Andrade, D. L. Oliveira
53. "The Role of Rosemary in Managing Gastric Disorders" - C. S. Martins, J. A. Salgueiro
54. "Rosemary Extracts and Their Efficacy in Gastric Mucosal Health" - F. L. Miguel, A. D. Cruz

COPYRIGHT & CREDITS	2
Prologue: A Guide to Wellness	3
INTRODUCTION	4
GASTRITIS	5
Symptoms	7
Types	9
Causes	13
Possible Long-Term Complications	16
Symptom Reduction and Prevention	18
Diagnostic Medical Tests	21
Warning Signs	23
FREQUENTLY ASKED QUESTIONS	25
124 FAQs about Gastritis	26
SUGGESTED PRACTICAL PLAN	42
NUTRITIONAL SUPPLEMENTS	44
Essential Precautions	45
Nutritional Supplements and Gastritis	45
Chamomile	45
Curcumin	46
Ginger	47
Glutamine	48
Licorice	49
Probiotics	50
Vitamin B12	51
Zinc	52
Strategic Supplement Combinations	53
Adverse Effects, Contraindications, and Interactions	54
Chamomile	54
Curcumin	55
Ginger	55
Glutamine	55
Licorice	55
Probiotics	56
Vitamin B12	56
Zinc	56
FOODS THAT TRANSFORM	57
Understanding the Link Between Nutrition and Health	58
Cooking Techniques	60
Tips to Prevent and Ease Gastritis	61
Healing Foods, according to TCM	63

Natural Remedies for H. Pylori ... 66
   Broccoli ... 66
   Ginger ... 66
   Lemon Verbena Essential Oil ... 66
   Licorice ... 67
Lemon and Gastritis: Myth or Remedy? ... 67
Beneficial Foods and Beverages ... 69
Harmful Foods and Beverages ... 70
Gastritis Support: Easy and Tasty Recipes ... 72
   Breakfast Options ... 72
   Lunch Creations ... 73
   Snacks ... 76
   Dinner Ideas ... 77

JUICES AND SMOOTHIES ... 81

Juices: Unleash Their Power ... 82
Homemade vs. Commercial Juices ... 84
Advantages of Homemade Juices ... 86
Possible Adverse Effects ... 87
When to Take Them ... 88
Preparation Tips ... 89
Key Recommendations ... 90
Nutritious Juice Recipes for Gastritis ... 92

MEDICINAL PLANTS ... 95

Essential Information ... 97
Guidelines for Care with Herbal Remedies ... 98
Medicinal Plants for Gastritis ... 98
   Aloe vera (Aloe barbadensis) ... 99
   Boldo (Peumus boldus) ... 99
   Chamomile (Chamaemelum nobile) ... 100
   Fennel (Foeniculum vulgare) ... 100
   Ginger (Zingiber officinale) ... 100
   Green Anise (Pimpinella anisum) ... 101
   Licorice (Glycyrrhiza glabra) ... 101
   Rosemary (Rosmarinus officinalis) ... 102
Phytotherapy Recipes ... 102
Learn Everything You Need to Know About the Plants ... 103
   Aloe vera (Aloe barbadensis) ... 104
   Boldo (Peumus boldus) ... 106
   Calendula (Calendula officinalis) ... 108
   Chamomile (Matricaria chamomilla) ... 110
   Fennel (Foeniculum vulgare) ... 112

Ginger (Zingiber officinale)	115
Green anise (Pimpinella anisum)	118
Lemon balm (Melissa officinalis)	120
Licorice or Liquorice (Glycyrrhiza glabra)	122
Mallow (Malva sylvestris)	125
Marshmallow (Althaea officinalis)	127
Rosemary (Rosmarinus officinalis)	129
Yarrow (Achillea millefolium)	131
BIBLIOGRAPHY & SCIENTIFIC STUDIES	**134**

www.ingramcontent.com/pod-product-compliance
Lightning Source LLC
Chambersburg PA
CBHW052303220526
45471CB00001B/465